食材性味与功效
编 委 会

主　编　柴可夫　　马　纲

编　委　（以姓名笔画为序）

　　　　王勇人　　牛永宁

　　　　孔明顺　　代民涛

　　　　李秀月　　谷英敏

　　　　钱俊文　　钱俊华

　　　　黄在委　　蒋剑锋

　　　　熊艳艳

主　译　蒋剑锋

译　者　（以姓名笔画为序）

　　　　张国利　　唐　路

The Characteristics and Effects of Food Ingredients

Chief Compiler   Chai Kefu   Ma Gang

Compiling Committee   (listed in the order of strokes of their Chinese name)

Wang Yongren	NiuYongning
Kong Mingshun	Dai Mindao
Li Xiuyue	Gu Yingmin
Qian Junwen	Qian Junhua
Huang Zaiwei	Jiang Jianfeng
Xiong Yanyan	

Chief Translator   Jiang Jianfeng

Translating Committee   (listed in the order of strokes of their Chinese name)

Zhang Guoli	Tang Lu

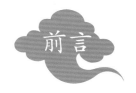

前言

　　食材是指烹制食物时所需、所用的原材料。我国幅员辽阔、地形复杂、气候多样，孕育着丰富的食材资源。自古以来便有"民以食为天"之说。炎黄子孙受大自然之馈赠，获取食材，使生命能够延续，从而使我中华民族得以繁衍不息。

　　在中医药理论指导下的饮食养生文化是祖国历史文化中的一颗璀璨的明珠。以食材之味，取药材之性，从而达到养生的目的。《内经·素问·脏气法时论》有言："五谷为养，五果为助，五畜为宜，五菜为充，气味合而服之，以补益精气。"唐代"药圣"孙思邈曰："食能排邪而安脏腑，悦神爽志，以资血气。若能用食平疴，释情遣疾者，可谓良工。"又曰："夫为医者，当须先洞晓病源，知其所犯，以食治之，食疗不愈，然后命药。"由此可见食疗养生的重要性。因此，我们申请了国家公益性行业科研专项项目《中国食材性味归经功效理论系统整理研究》（项目编号：200807012），对近600味食材进行了整理研究，并从中精选出250味，编撰了《中国食材考》，以供人们参考运用。

　　随着我国对外开放的深入，与国外的交流日益频繁，很多外国人士来到中国，对中国食物都是赞不绝口，百吃不厌。并常常随之对中国的饮食文化产生浓厚的兴趣。因此，我们在《中国食材考》的基础上，针对国外人士的饮食习惯以及对中国食物的喜好，从中挑选出120味食材，编撰了此书。书中主要介绍了每味食材的基原或来源、采收加工或制法、性味、归经、功用、服食方法、食宜食忌、储藏等内容，并配以彩图，图文并茂，以利于读者查阅。本书采用中英文对照的形式，以便于读者参考查阅。编者希冀此书能够对国内外民众的饮食生活产生积极的影响，并能够对中医食养文化在世界的弘扬与传播做出一点贡献。

　　由于编者水平所限，书中可能出现不妥之处，还请专家和广大读者提出宝贵意见。

Preface

Food ingredients in this book refer to materials that are needed and used when cooking food. China is a country with vast territory, complex terrain and various climates, and produces rich food resources. There is an old saying in China: "Food is what matters to the people". Chinese people receive food as gift from nature so that lives descend, and the nation sustains.

The diet health preserving culture under the guidance of TCM theories is a bright pearl in Chinese history and culture. Tasted as food, functioned as medicine, and health is preserved. *"Neijing·Suwen·Zangqifashilun"* has a saying: "Five grains as the main food, five animals as the supplement, five fruits and five vegetables as the complement, take the food when their nature and flavor are compatible, so as to tonify the essence and qi." The *"Herb Saint"* Sun Simiao in Tang Dynasty said: "Food can dispel evils and restore *Zangfu*, uplift spirit, so as to nourish blood and qi. It can be called a masterpiece if one can use food to relieve illness, calm the mood, and cure the disease." He also said: "As a doctor, one should have an insight to the origin of the illness, know its symptoms, and treat it by food. If food therapy doesn't work, then medication follows." All above shows the importance of diet health preserving. We applied a National Nonprofit Industries Scientific Research Project—"A Systematic Collection of Chinese Food Ingredients on the Theories of Nature, Flavor, Meridian Entry, and Function" (Project code: 200807012), we compiled 600 food materials and selected 250 of them to be published as *"Chinese Food Ingredients Study"*.

With the deepening of China's opening-up, international exchange has rapidly increased. Many foreigners come to China, and are deeply impressed by Chinese foods, which often grows their interests on Chinese food culture. Therefore, on the base of "Chinese Food Ingredients Study", considering foreign people's diet habits and their preference to Chinese foods, we selected 120 food ingredients to compile this book. The book mainly introduces the origin, collection/processing, flavor/properties, channels entered, function, indications, preparation/consumption, cautions/contraindications, and storage of each food ingredient, and we illustrated pictures to help reader to make reference. The book is written by a Chinese-English bilingual way to help reader to understand. We hope this book will have some positive influence on the diet of people both domestic and international, and make contribution to the spread of TCM diet health preserving culture to worldwide.

There might be something inappropriate in the book, so criticisms and corrections are warmly welcome.

谷豆类 Grains and Beans / 1

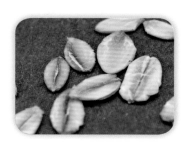

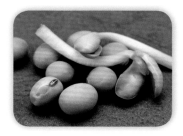

蔬菜类 Vegetables / 17

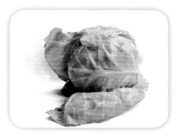

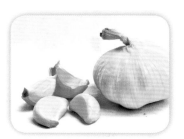

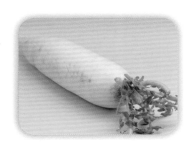

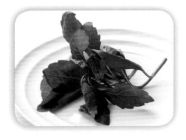

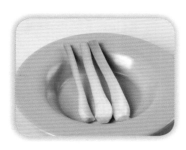

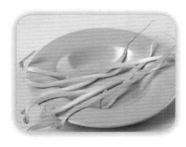

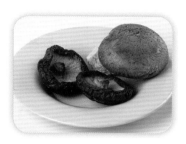

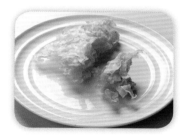

🍃 水果类 Fruits ／ 89

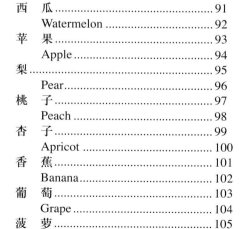

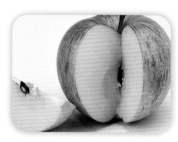

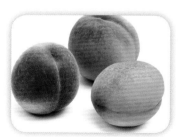

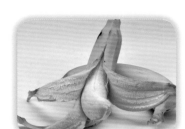

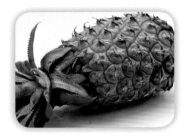

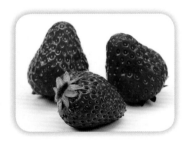

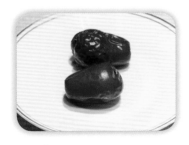

🐾 干果类 Dried Fruits / 149

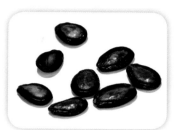

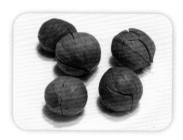

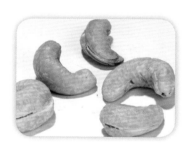

🐾 肉类 Meat / 173

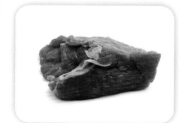

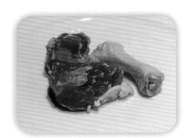

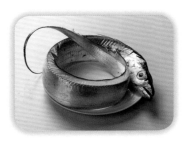

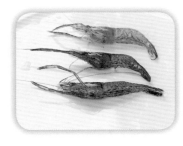

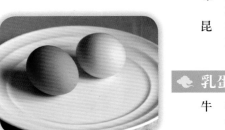

🌸 调味类 Seasonings ／ 221

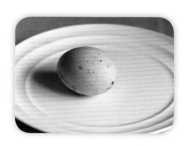

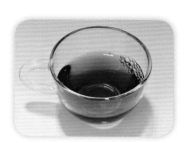

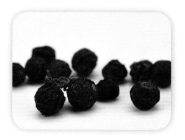

🌸 药食两用类 Herbal Foods ／ 241

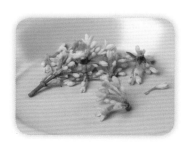

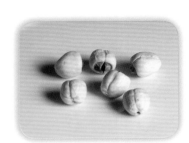

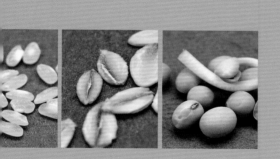

谷豆类

Grains and Beans

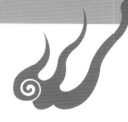

小 麦
Xiao Mai

【基原或来源】

为禾本科植物小麦*Triticum aestivum* L.的种仁。

【采收加工或制法】

夏季成熟时收割，脱粒后晒干贮藏或磨成面粉。购买时以麦粒饱满完整，黄棕色者为佳。

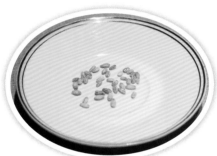

【性味】 性微寒，味甘。无毒。

【归经】 入心、脾、肾经。

【功用】

养心益肾，除热止渴，健脾止泻，敛汗通淋。适宜于各种人群，尤其是脏躁，烦热，虚汗，消渴，泄泻，乳痈，外伤出血，淋病，烫伤者食用。

【服食方法】

麦仁可煎汤饮用；面粉可煮粥、蒸馒头、烙饼、做手擀面等，也为饼干、面包、方便面等多种食品的原料；也是制作啤酒、酒精的常用原料。

【食宜食忌】

脾胃湿热者、小儿食积者慎食。民间有"麦吃陈，米吃新"的说法，存放时间长些的面粉比新磨的面粉的品质为好。

【储藏】

可盛放于密封容器内，置于阴凉、干燥、通风处。

Xiao Mai

Wheat

【Origin】
It is the kernel of *Triticum aestivum* L. of family Poaceae.

【Collection / Processing】
Collect the ripe fruit in summer. Thresh the seed and dry in the sun or grind into powder. The kernel which is plump and complete with yellowish-brown color is of good quality.

【Flavor / Properties】 Slight cold in nature, sweet in taste and non-toxic.

【Meridian Tropism】 Heart, Spleen and Kidney.

【Functions and Indications】
Nourish heart and tonify kidney, relieve heat and quench thirsty, invigorate spleen to check diarrhea, arrest sweating and relieve stranguria. It is suitable for all the people, especially those who have hysteria, dysphoria with smothery sensation, sweating due to debility, diabetes, diarrhea, acute mastitis, traumatic bleedings, stranguria, scalding, etc.

【Preparation / Consumption】
The kernel can be used to cook soup, the powder to cook porridge, make steamed bun, bake pancake, make handmade noodles, or be used as the raw material for making biscuit, bread, instant noodles, beer and alcohol, etc.

【Cautions / Contraindications】
The one who has dampness and heat in spleen or stomach, children with infantile indigestion due to food retention should take it with caution. As the saying goes:*Wheat is better to be consumed after storage,while rice before storage*. The folk people believe that the long-term preserved flour is better than the new-ground in quality.

【Storage】
Preserved in air-tight container in cool, dry and well-ventilated place.

燕 麦
Yan Mai

【基原或来源】

为禾本科植物燕麦*Avena fatua* L.的种仁。

【采收加工或制法】

夏季收割成熟果实，晒干后，去皮壳备用。购买时以颗粒完整、外表光润呈黄褐色者为佳。

【性味】味甘，性平。无毒。

【归经】入脾、大肠经。

【功用】

补虚，止汗，滑肠。适宜于久病体虚，纳差，便秘，自汗、多汗、盗汗等人食用。

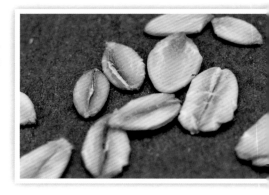

【服食方法】

煮粥，研末作面蒸饼，研末炒熟、开水冲调食，或加工成各种燕麦制品。

【食宜食忌】

肠滑易泻者慎食。

【储藏】

置于阴凉、干燥、通风处，防蛀防潮。

Yan Mai

Oat

【Origin】
The seed kernel of *Avena fatua* L., in the family of Poaceae.

【Collection / Processing】
Harvest mature fruit in summer, dry in the sun, and remove the peel and the shell for use. It is best to purchase the oats with full grain, smooth appearance and yellowish brown color.

【Flavor / Properties】 Sweet in flavor, neutral in nature, and non-toxic.

【Meridian Tropism】 Spleen and Large Intestine.

【Functions and Indications】
Tonify deficiency, suppress sweating, and lubricate intestine. Weakness due to long-term illness, poor appetite, constipation, spontaneous perspiration, hidrosis and night sweat.

【Preparation / Consumption】
It can be cooked congee, ground into powder to make steamed cake or to be fried, mixed in food with boiling water, or processed into various oat products.

【Cautions / Contraindications】
Those with intestinal smooth or diarrhea should be cautious to take it.

【Storage】
It should be put at shady, cool, dry and ventilate place, with moth proofing and moisture proofing.

粳 米
Jing Mi

【基原或来源】

　　为禾本科稻属植物稻（粳稻）*Oryza sativa* L.去壳的种仁。

【采收加工或制法】

　　秋季颖果成熟时采收，脱下果实，晒干，除去稻壳即可食用。购买时以外观完整、坚实、饱满、无虫蛀、无霉点、无异物夹杂者为佳。

【性味】 性平，味甘。

【归经】 入肺、脾、胃经。

【功用】

　　健脾和胃，补中益气，除烦渴，止泻痢。适宜于各类人群，尤其是脾胃虚弱，食少纳呆，倦怠乏力，心烦口渴，泻下痢疾者食用。

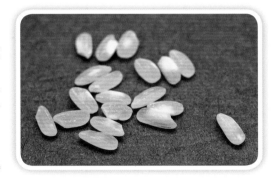

【服食方法】

　　可煮粥食用，也可加工成爆米花等食品。

【食宜食忌】

　　煮粥时不宜放碱，因其会破坏粳米中的维生素B_1，导致脚气病。

【储藏】

　　贮于干燥的有盖容器内，置于阴凉、干燥、通风处保存，以防虫蛀。

Jing Mi

Polished Round-grained Rice

【Origin】
It is the shelled seed of *Oryza sativa* L. of japonica rice of family Poaceae.

【Collection / Processing】
Collect the ripe caryopsis in autumn. Pick up the rice and dry in the sun. Remove the rice hull for consumption. The rice which is complete, solid, plump without damage by worms, mildew and impurities is of good quality.

【Flavor / Properties】 Moderate in nature and sweet in taste.

【Meridian Tropism】 Lung, Spleen and Stomach.

【Functions and Indications】
Invigorate spleen and harmonize stomach, tonify the middle energizer and invigorate *qi*, relieve polydipsia and diarrhea. It is suitable for all the people, especially for those who have deficiency of spleen and stomach, poor appetite and indigestion, lassitude and fatigue, vexation and thirsty, diarrhea and dysentery, etc.

【Preparation / Consumption】
Cook soup or process as popcorn, etc.

【Cautions / Contraindications】
It is unadvisable to put soda when cooking porridge because soda can ruin Vitamin B_1 in the rice and result in beriberi.

【Storage】
Preserved in a dry container with a cover in cool, dry and well-ventilated place to prevent from borer.

黄 豆
Huang Dou

【基原或来源】

为豆科植物大豆*Glycine max*（L.）Merr.的种皮黄色的种子。

【采收加工或制法】

秋季果实成熟后采收，取其种子晒干。

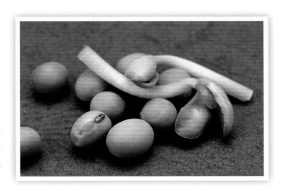

【性味】味甘，性平。

【归经】入脾、胃、大肠经。

【功用】

健脾利水，导滞通便，解毒消肿。适用于食积泻痢，腹胀纳食呆，脾虚水肿，疮痈肿毒者食用。

【服食方法】

煮食、炒食、制豆浆、做豆腐、磨粉制饼等。

【食宜食忌】

不宜多食，痛风患者不宜食用。

【储藏】

置阴凉干燥处，防潮防蛀。

Huang Dou

Soybean

【Origin】
It is the yellow seed of *Glycine max*(L.)Merr. of family Leguminosae.

【Collection / Processing】
Collect the ripe fruit in autumn and take the seed to dry in the sun.

【Flavor / Properties】 Sweet in flavor and moderate in nature.

【Meridian Tropism】 Spleen, Stomach and Large Intestine.

【Functions and Indications】
Invigorate spleen to promote water metabolism, remove stagnancy to relieve constipation, detoxicate and relieve swelling. Used for diarrhea due to stagnated food, poor appetite due to abdominal distention, edema due to spleen deficiency, carbuncle, etc.

【Preparation / Consumption】
Cook, stir-fry, make soybean milk or toufu, or grind into powder to make cake, etc.

【Cautions / Contraindications】
It should not be taken too much and the person who has gout should not take the bean.

【Storage】
It should be preserved in cool and dry place and prevented from moisture and moth.

绿 豆
Lü Dou

【基原或来源】

　　为豆科植物绿豆 *Phaseolus radiatus* L.的种子。

【采收加工或制法】

　　秋季果实成熟采收，晒干。

【性味】 味甘，性凉。

【归经】 入心、肝、胃经。

【功用】

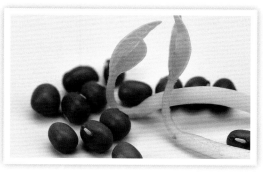

　　清热解毒，利水消暑。适用于中暑预防，暑热烦渴，水肿尿少，霍乱吐泻，风疹瘙痒，疮疡痈肿，药食中毒者使用。

【服食方法】

　　煎汤、煮食、生研绞汁或研末食用。

【食宜食忌】

　　胃寒者忌食。

【储藏】

　　置于阴凉干燥处，防蛀。

Lü Dou

Mung Bean

【Origin】
 It is the seed of *Phaseolus radiatus* L. of family Leguminosae.

【Collection / Processing】
 Collect the ripe seed in autumn and dry in the sun.

【Flavor / Properties】 Sweet in flavor and cool in nature.

【Meridian Tropism】 Heart, Liver and Stomach.

【Functions and Indications】
 Clear heat to detoxicate, promote water metabolism and relieve summer heat. Used for prevention of heatstroke, polydipsia due to summer heat, edema and oligurie, vomit and diarrhea due to cholera, itching skin due to rubella, carbuncles, medicine or food poisoning, etc.

【Preparation / Consumption】
 Decoct soup, cook, squeeze juice or grind into powder for consumption.

【Cautions / Contraindications】
 The one who has stomach cold should not take it.

【Storage】
 It should be preserved in cool and dry place and prevented from moth.

黑大豆
Hei Da Dou

【基原或来源】

为豆科大豆属植物大豆*Glycine max*（L.）Merr.的黑色种子。

【采收加工或制法】秋季果实成熟时采收，晒干。

【性味】味甘，性平。

【归经】入肾、脾、心经。

【功用】

补肾利水，调中下气，活血祛风，解毒消肿。适用于肾虚腰痛，水肿胀满，黄疸脚气，风痹痉挛，风痉口噤，痈肿疮毒，食物中毒者使用。

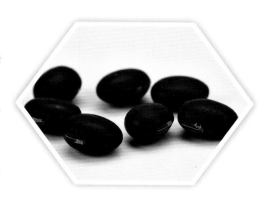

【服食方法】

煮食，炒食，捣粉作糕，捣汁饮等。

【食宜食忌】

脾胃虚弱者慎食。

【储藏】

置阴凉干燥处，防潮、防蛀。

Hei Da Dou

Black Soybean

【Origin】

It is the black seed of soybean plants of *Glycine max*(L.)Merr. in the family of Leguminosae.

【Collection / Processing】

Collect the ripe seed in autumn and dry the seed in the sun.

【Flavor / Properties】 Sweet in flavor and moderate in nature.

【Meridian Tropism】 Kidney, Spleen and Heart.

【Functions and Indications】

Tonify kidney and promote water metabolism, regulate the middle energizer and descend adverse *qi*, activate blood and expel wind, detoxicate and subside swelling. Used for lumbago due to kidney deficiency, edema and tumescence, jaundice and beriberi, spasm due to wind arthralgia, convulsion due to wind and trismus, carbuncles and poisonous sores, food poisoning, etc.

【Preparation / Consumption】

Cook, stir-fry, grind into powder to make cake or make juice.

【Cautions / Contraindications】

The one who has deficiency of spleen and stomach should take the soybean with caution.

【Storage】

Preserved in cool and dry place and prevented from moisture and moth.

薏苡仁
Yi Yi Ren

【基原或来源】

为禾本科薏苡属植物薏苡_Coix lacryma-jobi_ L.var._ma-yuen_（Romanet）stapf.的成熟种仁。

【采收加工或制法】

早熟种在大暑前后收获；晚熟种于霜降前后收获。待果实成熟后，采割全株，晒干后打下硬壳果实，再用碾米机碾去果壳及种皮，筛掉糠屑，收取种仁，再晒干后备用。购买时以颗粒完整饱满、色白、气味清新者为佳。

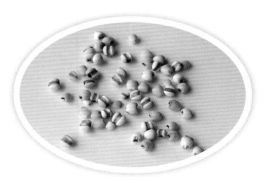

【性味】味甘、淡，性微寒。

【归经】入肺、脾、胃、肾经。

【功用】

健脾益胃，利水消肿，舒筋除痹，清热排脓。适宜于脾胃虚弱，食欲不振，水肿，喘息，淋病，脚气，泄泻，带下，风湿痹痛，筋脉拘挛，肺痈，肠痈，扁平疣者食用。

【服食方法】

可煎汤，煮粥，烧饭，炖羹，蒸食，做菜肴，酿酒，熬糖，磨成面粉用或加工成各种副食品等。

【食宜食忌】脾弱中气下陷者、大便难者及孕妇慎食。

【储藏】

宜贮藏于密封容器中，置放于阴凉、干燥、通风处，常翻晒，以防蛀防潮。

Yi Yi Ren

Coix Seed

【Origin】
It is the ripe kernel of *Coix lacryma-jobi* L. var.*ma-yuen*(Romanet)stapf.of family Poaceae.

【Collection / Processing】
The early maturing variety should be collected around Great Heat (12th solar term) while the late maturing variety around Frost's Descent (18th solar term). Collect the whole plant when the fruit is ripe, dry the plant and take the fruit with hard testa, remove the shell and testa by a rice mill and sieve the chaff crumbs to collect the kernel. Dry the kernel in the sun for consumption. The kernel which is complete and plump with white color and fresh odor is of good quality.

【Flavor / Properties】 Tasteless and sweet in taste, slightly cold in nature.

【Meridian Tropism】 Lung, Spleen, Stomach and Kidney.

【Functions and Indications】
Invigorate spleen and tonify stomach, promote water metabolism to relieve edema, sooth tendon to relieve pain, clear heat and discharge pus. Used for deficiency of spleen and stomach, poor appetite, edema, asthma, stranguria, beriberi, diarrhea, leukorrhea, pain due to wind and heat, spasm of tendons, lung abscess, intestine abscess, plane warts, etc.

【Preparation / Consumption】
Cook soup and porridge, stew thick soup, steam, make dishes, brew wine, boil sugar, grind into powder or process as subsidiary foodstuff.

【Cautions / Contraindications】
The one who has spleen deficiency with middle *qi* sinking, difficult bowel movement and the pregnant women should take it with caution.

【Storage】
Preserved in air-tight container in cool, dry and well-ventilated place. Bask it in the sun to prevent from moth and moisture.

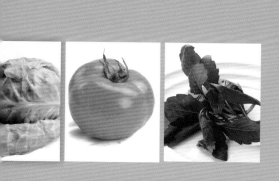

蔬菜类

Vegetables

白 菜
Bai Cai

【基原或来源】

为十字花科芸薹属植物大白菜*Brassica pekinensis* Rupr.的叶球。

【采收加工或制法】

秋、冬季采挖，除去泥土备用。选购时以叶球紧密严实、鲜嫩、无虫害者为佳。

【性味】 味甘，性平。

【归经】 入胃、膀胱大肠、小肠经。

【功用】

养胃止渴，利尿下气。适宜于脾胃不和、食积，热淋，便秘，丹毒，咽喉不利，喑哑，皮肤粗糙，气管炎，咳嗽，腮腺炎者使用。

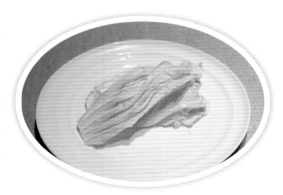

【服食方法】

可凉拌、炒食、做汤、做馅，腌制成泡菜，榨汁做饮料等。

【食宜食忌】

脾胃虚寒、大便溏泻者不宜多食。

【储藏】

用保鲜膜密封后放于冰箱保存；有条件者可置于地窖内贮藏。

Bai Cai

Chinese Cabbage

【Origin】
The leaf ball of *Brassica pekinensis* Rupr. in the family of Cruciferae.

【Collection / Processing】
Collected in autumn or winter, and ready for use after getting rid of the mud. Tips for purchase: it is advised to choose the one with tight leaf ball, fresh and tender, and no insect bites.

【Flavor / Properties】 Sweet in flavor and neutral in nature.

【Meridian Tropism】 Stomach, Bladder, Large Intestine and Small Intestine.

【Functions and Indications】
Nourish the stomach and quench thirst, diuresis and descends *qi*. Recommended for those with spleen-stomach disharmony, food accumulation, heat strangury, constipation, erysipelas, laryngopathy, loss of voice, pachycosis, tracheitis, cough or mumps.

【Preparation / Consumption】
It can be used for salad, stir-fried, made into soup, used as stuffing, pickled pickles , or juiced into beverage.

【Cautions / Contraindications】
Large quantity of consumption is not recommended for those with deficiency cold of the spleen and stomach or loose stool.

【Storage】
Sealed up with freshness-keeping plastic film to be stored in refrigerator. It can also be stored in cellar.

小白菜
Xiao Bai Cai

【基原或来源】

　　为十字花科芸薹属植物青菜*Brassica chinensis* L.的幼株。

【采收加工或制法】

　　四季皆可采收，以冬季者为上。选购时以菜体青翠，叶片完整者为佳。

【性味】味甘，性凉。

【归经】入肺、胃、大肠、小肠经。

【功用】

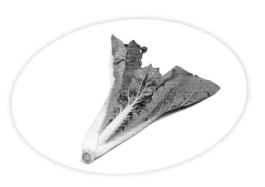

　　消食利肠，生津止渴，化痰止嗽。适宜于脾胃不和，食积，便秘，小便不利，消渴，心中烦热，肺热咳嗽，酒醉不醒，疮毒者使用。

【服食方法】

　　可凉拌，炒食，煮汤，腌渍，油炸，作火锅或麻辣烫配菜，榨汁做饮料等。

【食宜食忌】

　　素体脾胃虚寒易泄泻者慎食；服用甘草、白术、苍术等药者忌食。

【储藏】

　　保鲜膜密封，放于冰箱冷藏，可保存1周。

Xiao Bai Cai

Pakchoi

【Origin】

The young plant of *Brassica chinensis* L. in the family of Cruciferae.

【Collection / Processing】

It can be collected all year round, but those in winter is preferred. Tips for purchase: the one with green body and full leaf blades is better.

【Flavor / Properties】 Sweet in flavor and cool in nature.

【Meridian Tropism】 Lung, Stomach, Large Intestine and Small Intestine.

【Functions and Indications】

Promote digestion and benefits intestine, promote saliva production to quench thirst, resolve phlegm to stop coughing. Recommended for those with spleen-stomach disharmony, food accumulation, constipation, difficulty in micturition, wasting thirst, feverish dysphoria, cough with lung heat, drunkness, or sores.

【Preparation / Consumption】

It can be used for salad, stir-fried, boiled, pickled, or deep-fried, and it can also be used as side dishes for chafing dish, or squeezed to make juice.

【Cautions / Contraindications】

Use caution for those who are prone to have diarrhea due to deficiency cold of the spleen. Those who are using Licorice Root, Large-headed Atractylodes Rhizome or Swordlike Atractylodes Rhizome must not use it.

【Storage】

It can be stored in refrigerator for one week, sealed up with plastic wrap.

甘 蓝
Gan Lan

【基原或来源】

　　为十字花科芸薹属植物结球甘蓝*Brassica oleracea* L.var.*capitata* L.的球茎、叶。

【采收加工或制法】

　　全年皆可采收，春栽夏收称作夏甘蓝，夏栽秋收称作秋甘蓝。选购时以菜体完整、大小适中，无虫蛀、色泽鲜绿者为佳。

【性味】味甘，性平。

【归经】入胃、肾经。

【功用】

　　清热止痛，健胃补肾。适宜于胃及十二指肠溃疡，肾气不足，关节不利，失眠，头晕耳鸣，健忘，老年痴呆者使用。

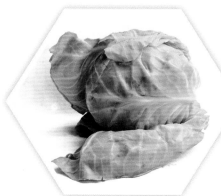

【服食方法】

　　可凉拌、炒食，做汤，做火锅配菜，腌制等。

【食宜食忌】

　　胃溃疡、胆囊炎等患者宜食；脾胃虚寒、泄泻者慎食。

【储藏】

　　放于阴凉、通风处或冰箱冷藏保鲜；亦可放地窖内贮藏。

Gan Lan

Broccoli

【Origin】
The corm and leaf of *Brassica oleracea* L. var. *capitata* L. of *Brassica* genus in the family of Cruciferae.

【Collection / Processing】
It can be collected all year round. The one planted in spring and harvested in summer is called summer kohlrabi, and the one planted in summer and harvested in autumn is called autumn kohlrabi. Tips for purchase: it is advised to choose the one with integrated shape, moderate size, no insect bites, and bright green color.

【Flavor / Properties】 Sweet in flavor and neutral in nature.

【Meridian Tropism】 Stomach and Kidney.

【Functions and Indications】
Expel heat to alleviate pain, invigorate the stomach and kidney. Recommended for those with gastric or duodenal ulcer, deficiency of kidney-*qi*, joints detriment, insomnia, dizziness and tinnitus, amnesia, or senile dementia.

【Preparation / Consumption】
Make salad, stir-fried, made into soup, used as side dishes for chafing dish, or pickled.

【Cautions / Contraindications】
Highly recommended for those with gastric ulcer or cholecystitis. Use with caution for those with deficiency-cold of spleen and stomach or diarrhea.

【Storage】
Stored in shady and ventilated area or cold-stored in refrigerator to keep freshness. It can also be stored in cellars.

黄 瓜
Huang Gua

【基原或来源】

　　为葫芦科植物黄瓜*Cucumis sativus* L.的果实。

【采收加工或制法】

　　夏季采收果实；鲜用。

【性味】味甘，性凉。无毒。

【归经】入肺、脾、胃经。

【功用】

　　清热利水，解毒利咽。用于热病口渴，咽喉肿痛，小便短赤，水火烫伤。

【服食方法】

　　生食、腌食、炒食、绞汁饮。

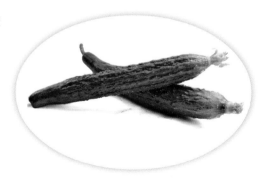

【食宜食忌】

　　脾胃虚寒者慎食。

【储藏】

　　放阴凉处保存。

Huang Gua

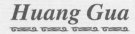

Cucumber

【Origin】
It is the fruit of *Cucumis sativus* L. of family Cucurbitaceae.

【Collection / Processing】
Collect the fruit in summer and take the fresh form.

【Flavor / Properties】 Sweet in flavor, cool in nature and non-toxic.

【Meridian Tropism】 Lung, Spleen and Stomach.

【Functions and Indications】
Clear heat and promote urination, detoxicate and relieve sore throat. Used for thirst due to febrile disease, sore throat, scanty urine in dark color, scalding.

【Preparation / Consumption】
Take the fresh fruit, or pickle, stir-fry, squeeze juice.

【Cautions / Contraindications】
The one who has deficiency-cold of spleen and stomach should take it with caution.

【Storage】
Preserved in cool place.

番 茄
Fan Qie

【基原或来源】

　　为茄科植物番茄*Lycopersicon esculentum* Mill.的果实。

【采收加工或制法】

　　夏、秋季果实成熟时采收，洗净，鲜用。

【性味】味甘、酸，性微寒。

【归经】入肝、肺、胃经。

【功用】

　　清热解毒，生津止渴，养血平肝，健胃消食。适用于咽干舌燥，烦热口苦，食欲不振，目糊不清，牙龈头晕，褥疮溃烂者使用。

【服食方法】

　　煎汤、煮粥、炒食、生食、绞汁服或做酱；外用：捣烂外敷。

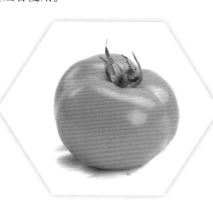

【食宜食忌】

　　大便溏烂者忌用。

【储藏】

　　放阴凉干燥处保存。

Fan Qie

Tomato

【Origin】
It is the fruit of *Lycopersicon esculentum* Mill. of family Solanaceae.

【Collection / Processing】
Collect the ripe fruit in summer and autumn, clean the fruit for fresh use.

【Flavor / Properties】 Sweet and sour in flavor, slightly cold in nature.

【Meridian Tropism】 Liver, Lung and Stomach.

【Functions and Indications】
Clear heat and detoxicate, generate saliva to quench thirst, nourish blood and sooth liver, invigorate stomach and promote digestion. Used for dry throat or parched tongue, vexation and bitter taste, poor appetite, blurred vision, gum bleeding, dizziness, bedsore, etc.

【Preparation / Consumption】
Make soup, cook porridge, stir-fry, consume the fresh fruit, squeeze juice or make ketchup. Mash the fruit for external use.

【Cautions / Contraindications】
It is contraindicated for the person who has loose stool.

【Storage】
Preserved in cool and dry place.

胡萝卜
Hu Luo Bo

【基原或来源】

为伞形科植物胡萝卜*Daucus carota* L.var. *sativa* Hoffm.的根。

【采收加工或制法】

冬季采挖根部，除去茎叶、须根，洗净。

【性味】味甘、微辛，性平。

【归经】入肺、脾经。

【功用】

健脾宽中，养肝明目，化痰止咳，清热解毒。用于食积脾虚，纳呆胃胀，痢疾泄泻，雀目眼花，咳嗽气喘，麻疹水痘。

【服食方法】

生食、炒食、煮粥、捣汁等。

【食宜食忌】

不宜多食。

【储藏】

放阴凉处保存。

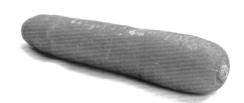

Hu Luo Bo

Carrot, Daucus Carota

【Origin】
The root of *Daucus carota* L.var.*sativa* Hoffm. in the Family of Apiaceae.

【Collection / Processing】
Collected the root in winter, and cooked after it has been cleaned and the stem, leaves, rootlets have been removed.

【Flavor / Properties】 Sweet and slightly acrid in flavor and moderate in nature.

【Meridian Tropism】 Lung and Spleen.

【Functions and Indications】
Strengthen spleen to soothe the middle, nourish liver to improve visual acuity, resolve phlegm to stop coughing, and clears away heat and toxic materials. Used to resolve food accumulation due to spleen asthenia, anorexia due to gastric distention, diarrhea due to dysentery, night blindness and dim eyesight, shortness of breath due to coughing, measles and chickenpox.

【Preparation / Consumption】
It can be eaten raw or be fried, boiled into porridge, or made into juice.

【Cautions / Contraindications】
Consumption of high quantities is not recommended.

【Storage】
Preserved in shady places.

莱 菔
Lai Fu

【基原或来源】

为十字花科莱菔属植物莱菔 *Raphanus sativus* L. 的鲜根。

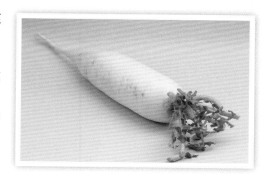

【采收加工或制法】

秋、冬季采挖鲜根，去掉茎叶，洗净。

【性味】生者味辛、甘，性凉；熟者味甘，性平。无毒。

【归经】入肺、脾、胃、大肠经。

【功用】

消积导滞，清热化痰，下气宽中，解毒止血。用于食积胀满，嗳腐吞酸，痢疾腹泻，痰热咳嗽，吐血，衄血便血，消渴失音，偏正头痛，烫伤，跌扑损伤。

【服食方法】

生食、捣汁饮、煮食、盐淹、晒干等。

【食宜食忌】

脾胃虚寒者不宜生食。

Lai Fu

Radish

【Origin】
　　It is the fresh root of *Raphanus sativus* L. of *Raphanus* plant of family Cruciferae.

【Collection / Processing】
　　Collect the fresh root in autumn or winter, remove the stem and leaves, clean for consumption.

【Flavor / Properties】 The raw radish is pungent and sweet in flavor, cool in nature, while the cooked radish is sweet in flavor, moderate in nature. Both the raw and the cooked are non-toxic.

【Meridian Tropism】 Lung, Spleen, Stomach and Large intestine.

【Functions and Indications】
　　Remove food retention and promote digestion, clear heat and resolve sputum, make *qi* flow downward and soothe the middle energizer, detoxicate and stop bleeding. Used for distention due to food retention, belching with fetid odour and acid regurgitation, dysentery and diarrhea, cough due to phlegmy heat, spitting blood, epistaxis, hemafecia, diabetes, aphonia, various headaches, scald and traumatic injury.

【Preparation / Consumption】
　　Take the fresh form, squeeze juice, cook, pickle or dry it in the sun.

【Cautions / Contraindications】
　　The one who has deficiency-cold of spleen and stomach should not take the raw radish.

大 蒜
Da Suan

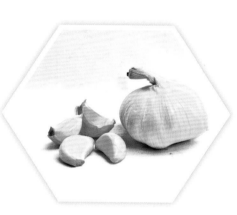

【基原或来源】

百合科葱属植物大蒜 *Allium sativum* L. 的鳞茎。

【采收加工或制法】

春、夏季采收，悬挂通风处，阴干备用。

【性味】味辛，性温，无毒。

【归经】入脾、胃、肺、大肠经。

【功用】

温中行滞，消肿散结，解毒杀虫。用于饮食积滞，脘腹冷痛，水肿胀满，泄泻痢疾，肺痨顿咳，痈疽肿毒，白秃癣疮，蛇虫咬伤以及钩虫蛲虫诸病。

【服食方法】

内食可煮食、煨食、生食、捣汁饮、制糖浆服或调味料用；外用：捣敷、贴敷、隔蒜灸、塞鼻、搐鼻或纳肛。

【食宜食忌】

热证，气血虚弱者，以及目疾、口齿、喉、舌诸患和时行病后均忌食或慎食。

【储藏】

置干燥通风处保存。

Da Suan

Garlic

【Origin】
The bulb of *Allium sativum* L. of *Allium* genus in the family of Liliaceae.

【Collection / Processing】
Harvested in spring and summer, and hung in ventilating places to be dried to be ready for use.

【Flavor / Properties】 Acrid in flavor, warm in nature, and nontoxic.

【Meridian Tropism】 Spleen, Stomach, Lung and Large Intestine.

【Functions and Indications】
Warm spleen-stomach to move stagnation, disperse swelling to remove nodulation, and neutralize poison to kill worms. Used to resolve food accumulation and stagnation, cold pain in the stomach duct and abdomen, distention and fullness due to edema, diarrhea due to dysentery, paroxysmal spasmodic cough due to tuberculosis, swelling and toxin of welling-abscess and flat-abscess, tinea tonsure lichen sores, bite wound of snake and worm, and diseases caused by hookworms and pinworm.

【Preparation / Consumption】
Internal use: It can be eaten raw, cooked by boiling, simmering, made into juice, syrup or seasoning. External use: It can be used for grinding application, paste application, garlic moxibustion, nostril-plugging therapy, nostril convulsion therapy, and anus admission.

【Cautions / Contraindications】
Those with heat zheng, *qi* and blood vacuity, and diseases of eyes, throat, and tongue, should avoid in eating or use with caution.

【Storage】
Preserved in dry and ventilating places.

生 姜
Sheng Jiang

【基原或来源】

为姜科植物姜*Zingiber officinale* Rosc. 的新鲜根茎。

【采收加工或制法】

秋季采挖，除去茎叶及须根，洗净泥土。

【性味】味辛，气温，无毒。

【归经】入肺、胃、脾经。

【功用】

发表散寒，温中止呕，化痰止咳，解诸毒。用于感冒风寒，恶寒发热，头痛鼻塞，寒痰咳喘，胃寒腹胀，呕吐泄泻，食鱼蟹及菌蕈等食物中毒。

【服食方法】

作调料、制腌姜、姜糖、榨汁等。

【食宜食忌】

疮痈热证及阴虚内热者忌服。

【储藏】

置阴凉潮湿处，或埋入湿沙内，防冻。

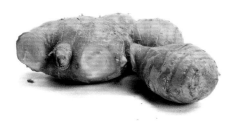

Sheng Jiang

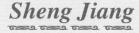

Ginger

【Origin】
The fresh rhizome of *Zingiber officinale* Rosc. of family Zingiberaceae.

【Collection / Processing】
Herborized in autumn. Remove the stems and leaves, wash the tuber.

【Flavor / Properties】 Pungent in flavor, warm in nature and non-toxic.

【Meridian Tropism】 Lung, Stomach and Spleen.

【Functions and Indications】
Disperse wind-cold, warm the middle energizer and arrest vomiting, resolve phlegm and stop coughing, detoxify various kinds of toxins. Used for common cold due to wind-cold, aversion to cold, fever, headache, stuffy nose, cough and asthma due to cold phlegm, abdominal distention due to cold in the stomach, vomiting, diarrhea or food poisoning caused by fish, crab and mushroom.

【Preparation / Consumption】
Can be made into seasoning, preserved ginger, ginger candy or juice, etc.

【Contraindications / Cautions】
Forbidden for the one who has sores and carbuncles of heat syndrome and internal heat due to *yin* deficiency.

【Storage】
It should be stored in cool and humid place, or buried in wet sand and prevented from frostbite.

菠 菜
Bo Cai

【基原或来源】

为藜科菠菜属植物菠菜*Spinacia oleracea* L.的茎叶。

【采收加工或制法】

冬、春季采收，除去泥土、杂质，洗净鲜用或晒干研末用。购买时以菜体鲜嫩翠绿、叶肥光亮、无虫蛀者为佳。

【性味】 味甘，性凉。

【归经】 入脾、胃、肝、大肠、小肠经。

【功用】

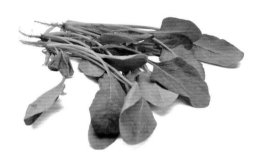

生津止渴，降气润肠，清肝明目。适宜于消渴引饮，便秘，痔疮出血，头痛目眩，风火赤眼，夜盲等人使用。

【服食方法】

煮食、捣汁、研末服、凉拌、炒食、做汤等。食前宜用开水焯一下，以破坏所含草酸，但不宜过久，以免维生素也被破坏。

【食宜食忌】

脾虚便溏者、肾病患者等慎食。

【储藏】

鲜品放阴凉处保存；干品放干燥处保存。

Bo Cai

Spinach

【Origin】

The stem and leaf of *Spinacia oleracea* L. of the genus of *Spinacia* in the family of Chenopodiaceae.

【Collection / Processing】

collected in winter or spring, remove the mud and foreign matters, used fresh after being cleaned or being grinded into powder after drying. It is advised to choose the one with fresh green body, bright colored and fleshy leaves, and no insect bites on purchasing.

【Flavor / Properties】 Sweet in flavor and cold in nature.

【Meridian Tropism】 Spleen, Stomach, Liver, Large Intestine and Small Intestine.

【Functions and Indications】

Promote the production of saliva to slake thirst, depress *qi* and moisten the intestines, clear the liver and brighten the eyes. Recommended for those with dispersion thirst with intake of fluid, constipation, bleeding from hemorrhoids, headache and dizziness, pathogenic wind-fire and acute conjunctivitis, or night blindness.

【Preparation / Consumption】

Boiled, made into juice, grinded into powder, salad, stir-fried, or made into soup. It is recommend to be blanched in hot water to destruct its oxalic acid, meanwhile, keep the process short to avoid the destruction of vitamins.

【Cautions / Contraindications】

Use caution for those with spleen asthenia and loose stool, or with nephrotic diseases.

【Storage】

Keep the fresh in shady and cool area, and the dried should be stored in dry area.

葱 白
Cong Bai

【基原或来源】

为百合科植物葱*Allium fistulosum* L.的鳞茎。

【采收加工或制法】

四季均可采挖，切去须根及叶，剥除外膜，晒干或鲜用。

【性味】味辛，性温，无毒。

【归经】入肺、胃经。

【功用】

发表通阳，解毒杀虫。适宜于感冒风寒，阴寒腹痛，二便不通，痢疾虫积，疮痈肿痛者食用。

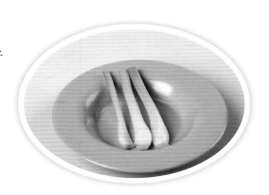

【服食方法】

生食、拌食、炒食、煮粥食、腌及作调味品等。

【食宜食忌】

表虚多汗者慎食。

【储藏】

干品密封保存，鲜品放置阴凉处。

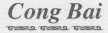
Cong Bai

Fistular Onion Stalk

【Origin】
　　The bulb of *Allium fistulosum* L.of Liliaceae Family.

【Collection / Processing】
　　Harvest in all seasons, and should be cooked fresh or be dried after the rootlets, leaves and outer layers have been removed.

【Flavor / Properties】 Acrid in flavor, warm in nature, and remove toxin and kill parasites.

【Meridian Tropism】 Lung and Stomach.

【Functions and Indications】
　　Effuse the exterior to activate yang, and remove toxin and kill parasites. Recommended for those with wind-cold common cold, abdominal pain due to *yin* cold, fecal and urinary stoppage, dysentery and intestinal parasitosis, or sore pain.

【Preparation / Consumption】
　　It can be eaten raw, mixed with other foods, fried, boiled into porridge, pickled or made into seasoning.

【Cautions / Contraindications】
　　Use caution for those with superficial asthenia and hyperhidrosis.

【Storage】
　　The dried should be sealed airtight, and the fresh should be preserved in shady place.

洋 葱
Yang Cong

【基原或来源】

为百合科葱属植物洋葱*Allium epa* L.的鳞茎。

【采收加工或制法】

于鳞茎外层鳞片变干时采收。选购时以其表皮干、包卷度紧、肉质细嫩、甜脆多汁者为好；从外表看，最好可以看出透明表皮中带有茶色的纹理。

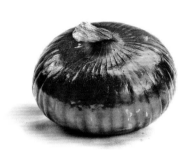

【性味】味辛、甘，性温。

【归经】入肝、脾、胃经。

【功用】

和胃理气，解毒杀虫，降压降脂。适宜于脾胃功能不佳，腹满腹胀、消化不良，食欲欠佳，滴虫性阴道炎，高血压、高血脂、动脉粥样硬化者使用。

【服食方法】

生食、凉拌色拉，烹炒、做汤、做馅食用，或作调味用。

【食宜食忌】

肥胖、高血压、高血脂者宜食。肺胃有热、眼目模糊者慎食。生洋葱不宜和蜂蜜同食。

【储藏】

置阴凉干燥处保存，防腐烂。

Yang Cong

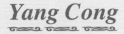

Onion

【Origin】
The bulb of *Allium epa* L. of *Allium* genus in the family of Liliaceae.

【Collection / Processing】
Collected when the flakes of the outer layer of the bulb turn to be dry. Tips for purchase: it is advised to choose the one with dry outer layers and tightly wrapped, tender in flesh, sweet and crisp in flavor, rich in juice. Superficially, it would be better if some tawny texture can be found in the transparent pericarp.

【Flavor / Properties】 Pungent and sweet in flavor, warm in nature.

【Meridian Tropism】 Liver, Spleen and Stomach.

【Functions and Indications】
Regulate stomach to smooth *qi*, remove toxin and kill parasites, lower blood pressure and fat. Recommended for those with spleen and stomach dysfunction, abdominal fullness and distension, dyspepsia, poor appetite, trichomonas vaginitis, hypertension, hyperlipemia, or atherosclerosis.

【Preparation / Consumption】
It can be consumed directly or used for salad, and it can also be stir-fried, boiled into soup, used as stuffing or seasoning.

【Cautions / Contraindications】
Highly recommended for those with obesity, hypertension or hyperlipemia. People with lung and stomach heat or vague vision should use with caution. The raw onion cannot be eaten together with honey.

【Storage】
Stored in shady, dry area to prevent being decayed.

茄 子
Qie Zi

【基原或来源】

　　为茄科植物茄*Solanum melongena* L.的果实。

【采收加工或制法】

　　夏、秋果熟时采收。

【性味】味甘，性凉。无毒。

【归经】入脾、胃、大肠经。

【功用】

　　清热消肿，活血止痛，宽肠利气。适宜于肠风下血，热毒疮痈，阴囊瘙痒，乳头裂破等人食用。

【服食方法】

　　可生食、凉拌、油炸、炒、烧、焖食、蒸、煮、做汤或干燥、腌菜食用。

【食宜食忌】

　　脾胃虚寒者勿食。

【储藏】

　　阴凉处保存。

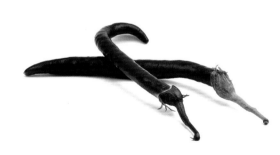

Qie Zi

Eggplant

【Origin】
The fruit of *Solanum melongena* L. in the family of Solanaceae.

【Collection / Processing】
Harvested in summer or autumn when it is ripe.

【Flavor / Properties】 Sweet in flavor, cool in nature, and nontoxic.

【Meridian Tropism】 Spleen, Stomach, and Large Intestine.

【Functions and Indications】
Clear heat and disperse swelling, promote blood circulation to arrest pain, broaden the intestines to induce *qi*. Recommended for those with intestinal wind bleeding, sores and abscess due to toxic heat, scrotum itching, or fissure of nipple.

【Preparation / Consumption】
It can be eaten raw, mixed with other food, cooked by being deep-fried, stir-fried, barbecued, stewed, steamed, boiled or made into soup. It can also be eaten after it has been dried or pickled.

【Cautions / Contraindications】
Contraindicated for those with deficiency-cold of spleen and stomach.

【Storage】
Preserved in shady place.

藕
Ou

【基原或来源】

　　为睡莲科植物莲*Nelumbo nucifera* Gaertn.的肥大根茎。

【采收加工或制法】

　　秋、冬及春初采挖。

【性味】味甘，性寒。无毒。

【归经】入心、脾、胃经。

【功用】

　　清热止血，凉血散瘀，生津止渴，健脾开胃，解酒止泻。用于热病烦渴，吐血衄血，热淋尿血，伤酒积食，泄泻痢疾。

【服食方法】

　　生食、捣汁或煮食。

【食宜食忌】

　　生食不宜过多。

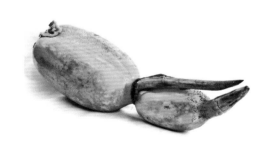

【储藏】

　　鲜品宜低温保存。

Ou

Lotus Root

【Origin】
It is the hypertrophic rhizome of *Nelumbo nucifera* Gaertn. of family Nymphaeaceae.

【Collection / Processing】
Collected in autumn, winter and early spring.

【Flavor / Properties】 Sweet in flavor, cold in nature and non-toxic.

【Meridian Tropism】 Heart, Spleen and Stomach.

【Functions and Indications】
Clear heat and stop bleeding, cool blood and resolve blood stasis, generate saliva to slake thirst, invigorate spleen to stimulate the appetite, disintoxicate and antidiarrheic. Used for polydipsia due to febrile disease, spitting blood or epistaxis, hematuria due to heat stranguria , sick due to overdrinking, indigestion, diarrhea and dysentery.

【Preparation / Consumption】
Fresh consumption is advised, or squeeze juice, boiled.

【Cautions / Contraindications】
Over-consumption should be avoided.

【Storage】
Fresh root should be preserved in low temperature.

旱芹
Han Qin

【基原或来源】

为伞形科芹属植物芹菜*Apium graveolens* L.的嫩茎叶。

【采收加工或制法】

夏、秋季采收，洗净鲜用或备用。

【性味】味辛、甘、微苦，性凉。

【归经】入肺、胃、肝、膀胱经。

【功用】

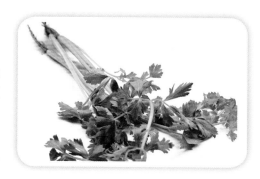

清热平肝，祛风利水，止血解毒。适宜于肝阳上亢所致高血压病，燥热心烦，肺热咳嗽，黄疸，乳糜尿，高血脂症，瘰疬，瘰疬，结核，跌打损伤所致瘀血肿毒，纳差，便秘，糖尿病，梅核气，饮酒过多，煤气中毒，肥胖者使用。

【服食方法】

可榨汁制作饮料，凉拌，炒食，煎汤，煮粥，腌制成泡菜等。

【食宜食忌】

脾胃虚寒易泄泻者不宜多食；不宜与黄瓜、鸡肉、鳖肉等同食。

【储藏】

可放于阴凉干燥处暂存；或用硅窗袋保鲜，在0~12℃可存放11天左右。

Han Qin

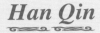

Celery

【Origin】
The young stem and leaf of *Apium graveolens* L. of *Apium* genus in the family of Apiaceae.

【Collection / Processing】
Collected in summer or autumn, make it clean and use fresh.

【Flavor / Properties】 Pungent, sweet and slightly bitter in flavor, cool in nature.

【Meridian Tropism】 Lung, Stomach, Liver and Bladder.

【Functions and Indications】
Clear heat and pacify the liver, dispel wind-evil and alleviate water retention, stop bleeding and resolve toxin. Recommended for those with hypertension caused by hyperactivity of liver *yang*, dysphoria due to dryness-heat, cough caused by lung-heat, jaundice, chyluria, hyperlipermia, rectal disease, scrofula, tuberculosis, ecchymoma caused by injuries from falls, poor appetite, constipation, diabetes, globus hystericus, excessive drinking, gas poisoning, or obesity.

【Preparation / Consumption】
It can be juiced to make beverage, cool-blended, stir-fried, boiled into soup, or pickled.

【Cautions / Contraindications】
Large quantity consumption is not recommended for those with deficiency cold of the spleen and who are prone to have diarrhea. It should not be taken together with cucumber, chicken or turtle meat.

【Storage】
It can be temporarily kept in shady and dry area, or placed in silicon window bags to keep freshness. The storage duration can be about 11 days with the temperature of 0°C~12°C.

青椒
Qing Jiao

【基原或来源】

为茄科植物青椒*Capsicum frutescens* var. *grossum*的果实。

【采收加工或制法】

秋季采收。采收前一周禁止喷洒农药。

【性味】 味辛、甘、微辣，性温。

【归经】 入心、脾、胃经。

【功用】

温胃消食，散寒除湿，通便，润肤。适宜于脾胃虚寒所致的胃痛、食欲不振、消化不良、痢疾、泄泻、畏寒肢冷、便秘，贫血，牙龈出血，身倦无力，皮肤干燥，冻疮，肌肉疼痛，癌症，肥胖者使用。

【服食方法】

可炒食，如青椒炒肉、青椒炒蛋等；也可做汤、做馅；也宜凉拌，如配以芹菜、洋葱等调拌。

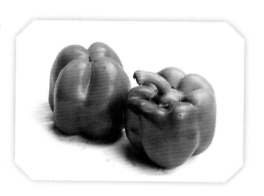

【食宜食忌】

青椒性温，患疮疡、糖尿病者慎食。

【储藏】

可放于阴凉、通风处或用保鲜膜包好放于冰箱暂存。

Qing Jiao

Green Pepper

【Origin】
The fruit of *Capsicum frutescens* var. *grossum* in the family of Solanaceae.

【Collection / Processing】
Collected in autumn. No pesticides one week before collection.

【Flavor / Properties】 Pungent, sweet and slightly spicy in flavor, warm in nature.

【Meridian Tropism】 Heart, Spleen and Stomach.

【Functions and Indications】
Warm the stomach and promote digestion, dispel cold and dampness, free movement of the bowels, and moisturize skin. Used for those with stomachache caused by deficiency-cold of spleen and stomach, poor appetite, dyspepsia, dysentery, diarrhea, cold limbs and fear of cold, constipation, anemia, gingival bleeding, fatigue, xerosis cutis, chilblain, myalgia, cancer, or obesity.

【Preparation / Consumption】
Stir-fried with meat or eggs, made into soup or stuffing, or used for salad, cool-blended with celery or onion for instance.

【Cautions / Contraindications】
For the warm nature, those with sores ulceration or diabetes should use with caution.

【Storage】
Stored in shady, ventilated area, or sealed up with freshness-keeping plastic bags to be stored in refrigerator.

山 药
Shan Yao

【基原或来源】

为薯蓣科薯蓣属植物山药*Dioscorea opposita* Thunb.的块茎。

【采收加工或制法】

秋、冬季采挖，挖时应注意，以免铲断。挖后洗净块茎泥土，储藏备用。

【性味】 味甘，性温。

【归经】 入心、肺、脾、肾经。

【功用】

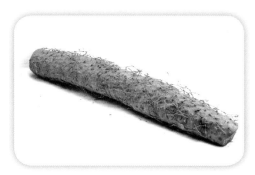

补脾益气，润肺化痰，强筋壮骨，安神益智。适宜于脾胃虚弱，泄泻，痢疾，咳嗽多痰，腰膝疼痛、筋骨不利，阳痿，遗精，失眠，智力低下，皮肤干燥，疮疡肿毒者食用。

【服食方法】

可煮粥，炒食，煲汤，凉拌，蒸食，山药汁可作茶饮，碾粉可蒸制糕点等。

【食宜食忌】

水肿、气滞患者慎食。

【储藏】

放于阴凉干燥处或冰箱冷藏，也可放于地窖内保存。

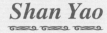

Shan Yao

Chinese Yam

【Origin】
It is the tuber of *Dioscorea opposita* Thunb. of family Dioscoreaceae.

【Collection / Processing】
Collect the tuber in autumn or winter. Pay attention when digging to prevent breakage of the tuber. Clean the tuber for consumption.

【Flavor / Properties】 Sweet in taste and warm in nature.

【Meridian Tropism】 Heart, Lung, Spleen and Kidney.

【Functions and Indications】
Tonify spleen and replenish *qi*, moisten lung to resolve phlegm, strengthen tendon and bone, tranquilize mind and promote intelligence. Used for deficiency of spleen and stomach, diarrhea, dysentery, coughing with much sputum, lumbago, unfavorable tendon and bone, impotence, spermatorrhea, insomnia, hypophrenia, dry skin, ulcers, carbuncles and poisonous swollen, etc.

【Preparation / Consumption】
Cook porridge, stir-fry, stew soup, mix with seasonings, steam, etc. The yam juice can be used to make tea and the yam powder can be used to make cakes.

【Cautions / Contraindications】
The one who has edema and *qi* stagnation should take it with caution.

【Storage】
Preserved in cool and dry place, or refrigerated in a freezer, or stored in the cellar.

绿豆芽
Lü Dou Ya

【基原或来源】

为豆科植物绿豆 *Phaseolus radiatus* L．的幼芽。

【采收加工或制法】

将种子浸毫，发出嫩芽。

【性味】味甘，性凉。

【归经】入心、肝、三焦经。

【功用】

清热解毒，利尿消暑。适用于暑热烦渴，小便不利，带下淋浊，眼目生翳，酒食中毒者食用。

【服食方法】

炒食，略焯后拌食，做馅，煮食或捣烂绞汁饮等。

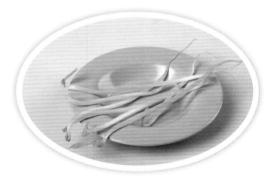

【食宜食忌】

胃寒者慎食。

【储藏】

放阴凉处保存。

Lü Dou Ya

Mungbean Sprout

【Origin】
It is the tender sprout of *Phaseolus radiatus* L. of family Leguminosae.

【Collection / Processing】
Immerse the mung bean to sprout.

【Flavor / Properties】 Sweet in flavor and cool in nature.

【Meridian Tropism】 Heart, Liver and Triple Energizer.

【Functions and Indications】
Clear heat and relieve toxicity, promote urination and relieve summer heat. Used for polydipsia due to summer heat, difficult urination, leukorrhea and turbid stranguria, nebula, food poisoning or alcoholism, etc.

【Preparation / Consumption】
Stir-fry, cook by scalding and mix with other food, make stuffing, or squeeze juice, etc.

【Cautions / Contraindications】
The one who has a cold in stomach should take it with caution.

【Storage】
It should be preserved in cool place.

苦 瓜
Ku Gua

【基原或来源】

　　为葫芦科植物苦瓜*Momordica charantia* L.的果实。

【采收加工或制法】

　　秋后采取，鲜用或切片晒干。

【性味】味苦，性寒。无毒。

【归经】入心、肺、脾、肝经。

【功用】

　　清暑止渴，明目，解毒。用于暑热烦渴、目赤疼痛、疮痈痢疾。

【服食方法】

　　可炒、煲汤或凉拌等食之。

【食宜食忌】

　　脾胃虚寒者，大便溏泄者慎食。

【储藏】

　　鲜者存放阴凉处，干品密封保存。

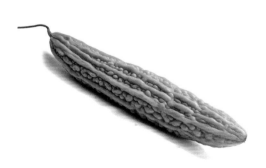

Ku Gua

Balsam Pear

【Origin】
It is the fruit of *Momordica charantia* L. of family Cucurbitaceae.

【Collection / Processing】
Collect the fruit after autumn, take the fresh form or slice it and dry it in the sun.

【Flavor / Properties】 Bitter in flavor, cold in nature and non-toxic.

【Meridian Tropism】 Heart, Lung, Spleen and Liver.

【Functions and Indications】
Clear summer-heat and quench thirst, improve eyesight, detoxicate. Used for vexation and thirst due to summer-heat, pink and painful eyes, sores and carbuncles.

【Preparation / Consumption】
Stir-fry, cook soup or mix with seasonings.

【Cautions / Contraindications】
The one who has deficiency-cold of spleen and stomach,or loose stool should take it with caution.

【Storage】
The fresh bitter gourd should be preserved in cool place while the dried material should be sealed air-tightly.

丝 瓜
Si Gua

【基原或来源】

　　葫芦科植物丝瓜*Luffa cylindrica* （L．） Roem．或粤丝瓜*Luffa acutangula*(L.) Roxb.的鲜嫩果实。

【采收加工或制法】

　　嫩丝瓜于夏、秋间采摘。

【性味】味甘，性微寒，无毒。

【归经】入肺、肝、胃、大肠经。

【功用】

　　清热化痰，凉血解毒，下乳通便，利尿消肿。用于身热烦渴，痰喘咳嗽，肠风下血，痔疮出血；血淋崩漏，乳汁不通，痈疽疮疡，疝气水肿。

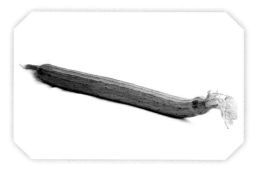

【服食方法】

　　可煮、炒食等。

【食宜食忌】

　　脾肾虚寒者慎食。

【储藏】

　　嫩丝瓜鲜用，阴凉处保存；老丝瓜晒干，干燥处保存。

Si Gua

Sponge Gourd

【Origin】
The fresh fruit of *Luffa cylindrica* (L.) Roem.or *Luffa acutangula*(L.) Roxb. in the family of Cucurbitaceae.

【Collection / Processing】
Harvest the immature sponge gourd in summer or autumn.

【Flavor / Properties】 Sweet in flavor, cold in nature, and nontoxic.

【Meridian Tropism】 Lung, Liver, Stomach, and Large Intestine.

【Functions and Indications】
Clear heat to resolve phlegm, cool blood to remove pathogenic heat, promote lactation and free the stool, induce diuresis to reduce edema. Used to resolve general fever and excessive thirst, phlegm panting and cough, discharging fresh blood stool, bleeding from hemorrhoids, blood stranguria ,metrorrhagia and metrostaxis, breast milk stoppage, carbuncle-abscess and sores ulceration, hernia and edema.

【Preparation / Consumption】
Boiled or fried.

【Cautions / Contraindications】
Use caution for those with deficiency-cold of spleen and stomach.

【Storage】
The immature should be used fresh, and preserved in shady place; the ripe should be dried, and preserved in dry place.

辣 椒
La Jiao

【基原或来源】

为茄科辣椒属植物辣椒*Capsicum annuum* L.的果实。

【采收加工或制法】

7～10月果实成熟时采收，鲜用或晒干用。

【性味】味辛，性热。

【归经】入心、脾、胃经。

【功用】

温中散寒，健胃消食。适宜于胃寒疼痛，脘胀厌食，呕吐泻痢，冻疮疥癣，风湿痹痛，风寒感冒等病症者使用。

【服食方法】

生食、炒菜、酿酒、做酱、用作火锅底料等。外用：适量，煎水熏洗、捣敷或取皮贴敷。

【食宜食忌】

阴虚火旺和痔疮、目疾者忌食。

【储藏】

鲜品放阴凉处保存，干品放干燥处保存。

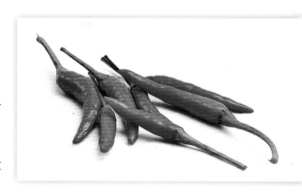

La Jiao

Hot Pepper

【Origin】
It is the fruit of *Capsicum annuum* L. of *Capsicum* plant of family Solanaceae.

【Collection / Processing】
Collect the ripe fruit during July to October, take the fresh fruit or dry it in the sun.

【Flavor / Properties】 Pungent in flavor and hot in nature.

【Meridian Tropism】 Heart, Spleen and Stomach.

【Functions and Indications】
Warm the middle energizer and disperse cold, invigorate stomach and improve appetite. Used for stomachache due to cold, epigastric distention, anorexia, vomiting, dysentery, chilblains, scabies, wind-dampness bi syndrome, common cold of wind-cold syndrome, etc.

【Preparation / Consumption】
Take the fresh fruit, stir-fried, brew wine, make sauce or the basic seasoning for hot pot. External use:Take appropriate amout, decocted into water for smoking or washing, or pounded for applying, or take the peel for patching.

【Cautions / Contraindications】
The one who has *yin* deficiency and excessive fire, hemorrhoids and eye problems should not take it.

【Storage】
The fresh pepper should be preserved in cool place and dried pepper in dry place.

莴 苣
Wo Ju

【基原或来源】

　　为菊科山莴苣属植物莴苣*Lactuca sativa* L.的茎、叶。

【采收加工或制法】

　　春季嫩茎肥大时采收，多为鲜用。

【性味】味苦、甘，性凉。

【归经】入胃、肝、肾经。

【功用】

　　清热解毒，利尿通乳。适宜于小便不利，或见尿血，乳汁不通，阴疝肿痛，虫蛇咬伤，疮疡肿毒等病症者食用。

【服食方法】

　　可凉拌，炒食，煮粥，腌制等。

【食宜食忌】

　　脾胃虚寒者忌食。

【储藏】

　　鲜品放阴凉处保存，干品放干燥处保存。

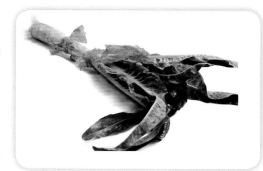

Wo Ju

Lettuce

【Origin】

It is the stem and leaf of *Lactuca sativa* L. of *Lactuca* plant of family Compositae.

【Collection / Processing】

Collect the fleshy tender stem in spring and it is usually taken in the fresh form.

【Flavor / Properties】 Bitter and sweet in flavor, cool in nature.

【Meridian Tropism】 Stomach, Liver and Kidney.

【Functions and Indications】

Clear heat and detoxicate, promote urination and active lactation. Used for difficulty urination, bloody urine, obstructed breast milk, swollen and sore due to hernia of *yin* syndrome, insect and snake bites, ulcers, carbuncles and poisonous swollen, etc.

【Preparation / Consumption】

Mix with seasonings, stir-fried, cook porridge and pickled.

【Cautions / Contraindications】

The one who has deficiency-cold of spleen and stomach should not take it.

【Storage】

The fresh stem is preserved in cool place and the dried stem in dry place.

冬 瓜
Dong Gua

【基原或来源】

为葫芦科植物冬瓜*Benincasa hispida*(Thunb.) Cogn.的果实。

【采收加工或制法】

夏末、秋初，果实成熟时采摘。去皮，洗净，去瓤食用。

【性味】 味甘、淡，性微寒，无毒。

【归经】 入肺、大小肠、膀胱经。

【功用】

清热祛暑，除烦，生津，化痰利水，解毒。适宜于暑热心烦，消渴，咳嗽痰喘，水肿胀满，淋证，脚气痛肿，泻痢痔漏，鱼毒酒毒，颜面色斑及肥胖者食用。

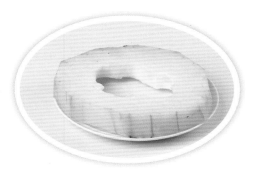

【服食方法】

煮汤，煨食，做药膳，捣汁饮；外用：捣敷或煎水洗。

1.《本草经集注》："直捣，绞汁服之。"

2.《本草衍义》："冬月收为菜，压去汁，蜜煎代果。患发背及一切痈疽，削一大块，置疮上，热则易之，分败热毒气甚良。"

【食宜食忌】

脾肾虚寒滑泄者慎食。

【储藏】

阴凉通风处保存。

Dong Gua

Wax Gourd

【Origin】
It is the fruit of *Benincasa hispida*(Thunb.) Cogn in the family of Cucurbitaceae.

【Collection / Processing】
Herborized during later summer and early autumn when the fruit is ripe. Peel the fruit and clean it, take it after removing the melon pulp.

【Flavor / Properties】 Sweet and tasteless in flavor, slightly cold in nature and non-toxic.

【Meridian Tropism】 Lung, Large Intestine, Small Intestine and Bladder.

【Functions and Indications】
Clear summer-heat, relieve restlessness, generate body fluid, resolve phlegm and promote diuresis and detoxicate. It is suitable for the one who has vexation due to summer-heat, diabetes, cough and asthma with sputum, edema and distension, stranguria, beriberi, carbuncles, diarrhea, anal fistula, toxicosis by fish and shrimp, alcoholism, color mottle on the face and the overweight.

【Preparation / Consumption】
For oral taking, make soup or cook it over a slow fire, make herbal cuisine or squeeze juice; For external use, smash it for topical application or decoct it to wash.

1. Annotated Shen Nong's Herbal: Smash it directly and squeeze juice.

2. Amplification on Materia Medica: Collected in winter as vegetable, squeeze the juice and decoct the remainder with honey as preserved fruit. For the patient who has carbuncle on the back or any other ulcers, cut a bulk to put on the ulcer. Remove it when it gets heated. It is quite good for relieving pyrotoxin.

【Contraindications / Cautions】
The one who has diarrhea due to deficient cold of spleen and kidney should take it with caution.

【Storage】
It should be preserved in shady, cool and well-ventilated place.

南 瓜
Nan Gua

【基原或来源】

为葫芦科植物南瓜*Cucurbita moschata* (Duch.ex Lam.)Duch.ex Poir.的果实。

【采收加工或制法】

夏、秋果实成熟时采收。

【性味】味甘，性温。

【归经】入肺、脾、胃经。

【功用】

补中益气，解毒消肿。适宜于脾虚气弱、营养不良，肺痈咯脓痰，烫伤及痈肿等人用之。

【服食方法】

炒、煮、蒸、做饼、做馅等食之。

【食宜食忌】

凡患气滞湿阻之病，忌食。

【储藏】

放阴凉处保存。

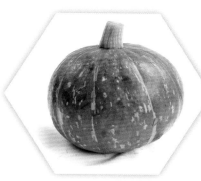

Nan Gua

Pumpkin

【Origin】

It is the fruit of *Cucurbita moschata* (Duch.ex Lam.)Duch.ex Poir. of family Cucurbitaceae.

【Collection / Processing】

Collect the ripe fruits in summer and autumn.

【Flavor / Properties】 Sweet in flavor and warm in nature.

【Meridian Tropism】 Lung, Spleen and Stomach.

【Functions and Indications】

Tonify middle energizer and benefit *qi*, detoxicate and eliminate swelling. Used for feeble *qi* due to spleen deficiency, malnutrition, purulent sputum due to lung abscess, scald, carbuncles and swelling, etc.

【Preparation / Consumption】

Stir-fry, cook, steam, make cake or stuffing for consumption,etc.

【Cautions / Contraindications】

The one who has *qi* stagnation and dampness obstruction should not take it.

【Storage】

Preserved in cool place.

韭 菜
Jiu Cai

【基原或来源】

为百合科植物韭菜*Allium tuberosum* Rottl.ex Spreng.的叶。

【采收加工或制法】

四季可采，鲜用。

【性味】味辛，性温。

【归经】入肝、肾、胃经。

【功用】

温阳补虚，行气理血，下气降逆，解毒散结，通腑利肠。用于腰膝酸冷，阳痿遗精，胸痹急痛，吐血唾血，衄血尿血，痔漏脱肛，反胃噎膈，痢疾便秘，跌打损伤，瘀血肿痛。

【服食方法】

炒食、凉拌、作馅、煮粥、作羹、捣汁饮等。外用：可煎汤熏洗，或热敷。

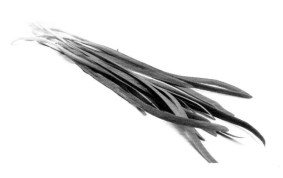

【食宜食忌】

阴虚火旺及患疮疡、目疾者慎食。

【储藏】

放阴凉处保存。

Jiu Cai

Leek

【Origin】
It is the leaf of *Allium tuberosum* Rottl.ex Spreng. of family Liliaceae.

【Collection / Processing】
It can be collected in any season and fresh consumption is advised.

【Flavor / Properties】 Pungent in flavor and warm in nature.

【Meridian Tropism】 Liver, Kidney and Stomach.

【Functions and Indications】
Warm yang and tonify deficiency, move *qi* and regulate blood, check adverse rise of *qi* and drive it downward, detoxicate and eliminate nodule, promote the movement of bowels. Used for aching waist and knee, impotence and emission,chest impediment and cramping pain, spitting blood, bloody urine and non-traumatic bleeding, hemorrhoid and rectocele, regurgitation and choked esophagus, dysentery and constipation, traumatic injury, swelling and pain due to blood stasis.

【Preparation / Consumption】
Stir-fry, mix with seasonings, make stuffings, cook porridge, make thick soup or squeeze juice. For external use, it can be cooked for fumigation-washing or hot compress.

【Cautions / Contraindications】
The one who has *yin* deficiency with effulgent fire, ulcer and eye disease should take it with caution.

【Storage】
Preserved in cool place.

西葫芦
Xi Hu Lu

【基原或来源】

为葫芦科南瓜属植物西葫芦*Cucurbita pepo* L.的果实。

【采收加工或制法】

春季或秋季播种，约50天后即可采收果实。选购时以表皮完整无损、色泽光鲜、果肉较多者为佳。

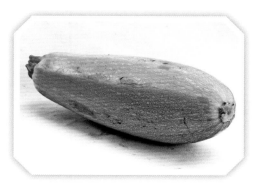

【性味】味甘、淡，性凉。

【归经】入肺、肾、膀胱经。

【功用】

清热利尿，润肺止咳，消肿散结。适宜于烦躁不寐，肺燥咳嗽，热淋，水肿，肾炎，热性便秘，肝硬化腹水，皮肤粗糙干燥者食用。

【服食方法】

可配以鸡蛋、西红柿、肉类等炒食；亦可做汤、作馅、煮粥等。烹调时不宜煮太烂，以免损失营养成分。

【食宜食忌】

不宜生食；夜盲患者宜食。

【储藏】

宜放于阴凉、通风处暂存或冰箱冷藏。

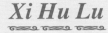
Xi Hu Lu

Zucchini

【Origin】
　　The fruit of *Cucurbita pepo* L. of Cucurbita in the family of Cucurbitaceae.

【Collection / Processing】
　　Planted in spring or autumn, and collected after about 50 days. Tips for purchase: it is preferred to choose the one with intact skin, bright color and more flesh.

【Flavor / Properties】 Sweet and bland in flavor, cool in nature.

【Meridian Tropism】 Lung, Kidney and Large Intestine.

【Functions and Indications】
　　Reduce fever and diuresis, moisten lung to stop cough, cure swelling and dissipate nodulation. Recommended for those with sleeplessness due to dysphoria, cough due to lung dryness, heat strangury, edema, nephritis, febrile constipation, cirrhosis ascites, or pachycosis.

【Preparation / Consumption】
　　It can stir-fried together with eggs, tomatoes, or meat. It can also be made into soup, porridge, or used as stuffing. To keep the nutrients, it is not advised to be boiled for too long.

【Cautions / Contraindications】
　　The raw one is not advised for consumption. It is recommended for people with night blindness.

【Storage】
　　Temporarily kept in shady and ventilated area, or it can be cold-stored in refrigerator.

雪里蕻
Xue Li Hong

【基原或来源】

为十字花科芸薹属植物分蘖芥*Brassica juncea* var.*multiceps* Tsen et Lee的嫩茎叶。

【采收加工或制法】

分春、冬两季。春季一般在3~4月采收；冬季在小雪前后采收。选购时以色泽鲜绿、脆嫩、无异味者为佳。

【性味】 味甘、辛，性温。

【归经】 入肺、胃、肝经。

【功用】

宣肺祛痰，开胃消食，温中利气，明目利膈。适宜于胸膈满闷，咳嗽痰多，食欲不振，疮痈肿痛，耳目失聪，牙龈肿烂，便秘者使用。

【服食方法】

可清炒或配以肉末、肉丝炒食；可做汤，如雪菜豆腐汤；也可做馅，腌制等。

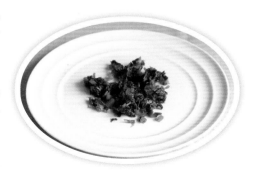

【食宜食忌】

慢性支气管炎属寒痰内盛者、纳差者、胸闷不舒者宜食；阴虚火旺者慎食。

【储藏】

鲜者可暂放冰箱冷藏；也可腌制后保存。

Xue Li Hong

Potherb Mustard

【Origin】
The young stem and leaf of *Brassica juncea* var.*multiceps* Tsen et Lee of *Brassica* genus in the family of Cruciferae.

【Collection / Processing】
It can be harvested in two seasons: spring and winter. In spring, it is usually around March to April, and in winter, it is usually around Slight Snow (20th solar term). Tips for purchase: it is advised to choose the one with bright green color, tender quality, and no peculiar smell.

【Flavor / Properties】 Sweet and pungent in flavor, warm in nature.

【Meridian Tropism】 Lung, Stomach and Liver.

【Functions and Indications】
Ventilate lung and expel phlegm, increase appetite and promote digestion, warm the middle energizer and remove *qi*, improve eyesight and benefit the diaphragm. Recommended for those with fullness and oppression in the chest and diaphragm, cough with excessive phlegm, poor appetite, ulcer and sore pain, loss of hearing and seeing, swollen gingiva, or constipation.

【Preparation / Consumption】
It can be stir-fried alone or with other foods such as meet, boiled into soup, used as stuffing, or pickled.

【Cautions / Contraindications】
Highly recommended for those with chronic bronchitis (exuberant internal phlegm-cold type), anorexia, or chest discomfort. Use caution for those with excessive pyrexia caused by *yin* deficiency.

【Storage】
The fresh can be temporarily kept in refrigerator, or it can be pickled for storage.

茭 白
Jiao Bai

【基原或来源】

　　为禾本科菰属植物菰*Zizania caduciflora* (Turcz.ex.Trin.) Hand.-Mazz.的嫩茎经菰黑粉菌的刺激而形成的纺锤形肥大的菌瘿。

【采收加工或制法】

　　夏、秋季采收，剥去叶片，洗净鲜用或晒干备用。

【性味】味甘，性寒。

【归经】入肺、肝、脾、胃经。

【功用】

　　清热解毒，除烦止渴，利尿通便。适宜于烦热消渴，二便不通，黄疸目赤，痢疾热淋，乳汁不下，酒精中毒，疮疡肿毒等病症者食用。

【服食方法】

　　凉拌、炒食、蒸、炖、煮汤等。

【食宜食忌】

　　脾虚泄泻者慎食。

【储藏】

　　鲜品放阴凉处保存，干品放干燥处保存。

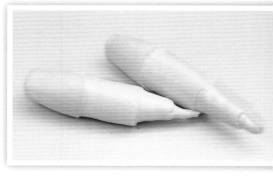

Jiao Bai

Wild Rice Stem

【Origin】
The fusiform fat fungus gall which comes, through the stimulation of ustilagomaydis, from the immature stem of *Zizania caduciflora* (Turez.ex.Trin.) Hand.-Mazz. of *Zizania* genus in the family of poaceae.

【Collection / Processing】
Collect in summer and autumn. Peel the leaves, clean the stem and dry it in the sun.

【Flavor / Properties】 Sweet in flavor and cold in nature.

【Meridian Tropism】 Lung, Liver, Spleen and Stomach.

【Functions and Indications】
Clear heat to detoxicate, relieve restlessness and thirst, promote urination and relax bowels. Used for vexation and diabetes, inability of urination and defecation, jaundice, conjunctival congestion, dysentery, stranguria due to heat, obstructed breast milk, alcoholism, ulcers carbuncles and poisonous swollen, etc.

【Preparation / Consumption】
Mix with seasonings, stir-fried, steam, stew and cook soup.

【Cautions / Contraindications】
The one who has diarrhea due to spleen deficiency should take it with caution.

【Storage】
The fresh fungus gall should be preserved in cool place and the dried fungus gall in dry place.

金针菇
Jin Zhen Gu

【基原或来源】

为白蘑科金针菇属金针菇*Flammulina velutipes*(Curt.ex Fr.)Sing.的子实体。

【采收加工或制法】

全年皆可栽培，尤宜在秋冬、早春时栽培，栽培10天后即可适时采集。选购时以新鲜、无异味者为佳。

【性味】 味甘、咸，性凉。

【归经】 入肝、胃经。

【功用】

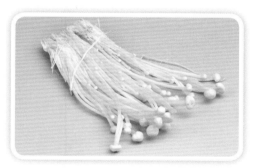

益胃利肝，增智抗癌。适宜于久病或术后体虚，习惯性便秘，高血脂，高血压，肝炎，胃及十二指肠溃疡，小儿生长缓慢，小儿弱智，老年性痴呆，癌症者使用。

【服食方法】

可凉拌，清炒，煮汤，也可作火锅及麻辣烫的原料。

【食宜食忌】

因性凉，脾虚易泄泻、腹痛者慎食。

【储藏】

用保鲜膜封好，放于冰箱冷藏。

Jin Zhen Gu

Enoki Mushroom

【Origin】

The fruiting body of *Flammulina velutipes* (Curt. ex Fr.) Sing. of *Flammulina* genus in the family of Tricholomataceae.

【Collection / Processing】

It can be cultivated all year round, especially in autumn, winter and early spring. It can be collected 10 days after cultivation. It is advised to choose the fresh one without peculiar smell.

【Flavor / Properties】 Sweet and salty in flavor, cold in nature.

【Meridian Tropism】 Liver and Stomach.

【Functions and Indications】

Benefit the stomach and liver, improve intelligence and prevent cancer. Recommended for those with weakness due to chronic disease or after operation, habitual constipation, hyperlipemia and hypertension, hepatitis, gastric and duodenal ulcer, stunt or mental retardation for children, senile dementia, or cancer.

【Preparation / Consumption】

It can be used for salad, stir-fried, boiled, or used as ingredients for chafing dish.

【Cautions / Contraindications】

For it cold nature, people who are prone to have diarrhea or abdominal pain due to spleen asthenia should use with caution.

【Storage】

Sealed up with freshness-keeping plastic film to be cold-stored in refrigerator.

金针菜
Jin Zhen Cai

【基原或来源】

为百合科萱草属植物黄花菜*Hemerocallis citrina* Baroni、萱草*Hemerocallis fulva*(L.)L.等的花蕾。

【采收加工或制法】

春夏花将开放时采收，鲜用，或直接晒干，或蒸后晒干。

【性味】 味甘，性凉。

【归经】 入心、肺、脾经。

【功用】

利湿解毒，宽胸解郁，清心安神。适宜于胸闷心烦，夜难安寐，小便短涩，黄疸尿赤，疮疡肿毒等病症者食用。

【服食方法】

凉拌、炒、熘、做汤等。

【食宜食忌】

脾虚便溏者慎食。

【储藏】

鲜品放阴凉处保存，干品放干燥处保存。

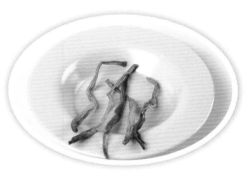

Jin Zhen Cai

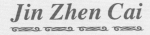

Daylily

【Origin】
It is the flower bud of *Hemerocallis citrina* Baroni and *Hemerocallis fulva*(L.) L. of family Liliaceae.

【Collection / Processing】
Collect the flower in spring or summer when it is going to bloom, take the fresh flower or dry it in the sun directly or after being steamed.

【Flavor / Properties】 Sweet in flavor and cool in nature.

【Meridian Tropism】 Heart, Lung and Spleen.

【Functions and Indications】
Promote urination and detoxicate, relieve chest distress and depression, clear heart heat and tranquilize mind. Used for chest oppression and vexation, poor sleep, little and painful urination, jaundice, dark urine, ulcers,carbuncles and poisonous swollen, etc.

【Preparation / Consumption】
Mix with seasonings, stir-fried, quick-fried or cook soup.

【Cautions / Contraindications】
The one who has loose stool due to spleen deficiency should take it with caution.

【Storage】
The fresh flower should be preserved in cool place and the dried flower in dry place.

茼 蒿
Tong Hao

【基原或来源】

为菊科茼蒿属植物茼蒿*Chrysanthemum coronarium* L.的嫩茎叶。

【采收加工或制法】

冬、春、夏季皆可采收，洗净备用。购买时以菜体清洁完整，茎壮叶肥，色泽鲜绿，无黄叶者为佳。

【性味】味辛、甘，性平。

【归经】入心、脾、胃经。

【功用】

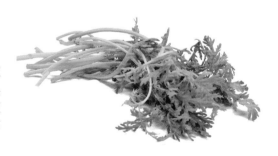

养胃安心，消痰行气。适宜于脾胃不和、消化不良，膈中臭气，心烦不安，咳嗽痰多，小便不利，便秘，疝气腹痛，肝气不舒，感冒、气管炎者使用。

【服食方法】

可凉拌，炒食，涮食，余汤，做馅，制作饮料等。

【食宜食忌】

脾胃虚寒者不宜多食。

【储藏】

用保鲜膜密封后，置于冰箱冷藏保鲜。

Tong Hao

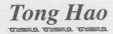

Crown Daisy

【Origin】

It is the tender stem and leaves of *Chrysanthemum coronarium* L. of family Compositae.

【Collection / Processing】

Collect it in winter, spring and summer, clean it for consumption. The plant which is clean and complete with strong stem, plump leaves in fresh green, and without yellow leaves is of good quality.

【Flavor / Properties】 Pungent and sweet in flavor, moderate in nature.

【Meridian Tropism】 Heart, Spleen and Stomach.

【Functions and Indications】

Nourish stomach and tranquilize heart, eliminate phlegm and promote *qi* movement. Used for disharmony of spleen and stomach, indigestion, belching with halitosis, vexation, coughing with much phlegm, difficult urination, constipation, abdominal pain due to hernia, obstructed liver *qi*, common cold, bronchitis, etc.

【Preparation / Consumption】

Salad, stir-fry, instantly boil, cook soup, make stuffings or drinks, etc.

【Cautions / Contraindications】

The one who has deficient cold of spleen and stomach should not consume it too much.

【Storage】

Preserved in a refrigerator after being sealed air-tightly with freshness protection package.

马 兰
Ma Lan

【基原或来源】

为菊科马兰属植物马兰*Kalimeris indica*（L.）Sch.-Bep.的嫩茎叶。

【采收加工或制法】

3～4月采摘嫩茎叶，洗净，鲜用或晒干备用。购买时以叶体较大、色泽鲜绿、气味清香者为佳。

【性味】味辛，性凉。

【归经】入肺、胃、肝、肾、大肠经。

【功用】

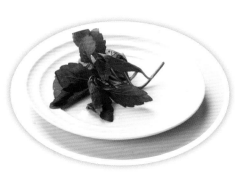

清热利湿，解毒消肿，凉血止血。适宜于感冒咳嗽，咽喉肿痛，痔疮淋浊，黄疸水肿，吐血衄血，血痢崩漏，创伤出血，丹毒蛇伤，小儿疳积等病症者使用。

【服食方法】

凉拌、炒食、做馅、煮汤或煎水代茶饮。食前需经沸水焯过，再用凉水清洗数遍，以去除苦涩之味。

【食宜食忌】

脾虚宜便溏者、孕妇慎食。

【储藏】

宜用保鲜袋密封，放阴凉、干燥处保存，或冰箱冷藏。

Ma Lan

Indian Kalimeris Herb

【Origin】
It is the tender stem and leaf of *Kalimeris indica* (L.)Sch.-Bep. of *Kalimeris* plant of family Compositae.

【Collection / Processing】
Collect the tender stem and leaves in March and April, clean it for fresh use or dry it in the sun. The plant with large leaves and fresh scent and jade green in color is superior in quality.

【Flavor / Properties】 Pungent in flavor and cool in nature.

【Meridian Tropism】 Lung, Stomach, Liver, Kidney and Large Intestine.

【Functions and Indications】
Clear heat and promote urination, detoxicate and relieve swollen, cool blood and stop bleeding. Used for coughing due to common cold, swollen and sore throat, hemorrhoids, turbid urination due to stranguria, jaundice, edema, vomiting blood, epistaxis, dysentery with blood, metrorrhagia and metrostaxis, traumatic bleeding, erysipelas, snake bites, infantile malnutrition, etc.

【Preparation / Consumption】
Mix with seasonings, stir-fried, make stuffings, cook soup, make tea. Before consumption, it should be put in boiling water and taken out immediately, wash with cool water several times to remove the bitter taste.

【Cautions / Contraindications】
The one who has loose stool due to spleen deficiency and the pregnant women should take it with caution.

【Storage】
Preserved in freshness protection package air-tightly and put in cool and dry place, or it can be refrigerate.

香 菇
Xiang Gu

【基原或来源】

为白蘑科香菇属真菌香菇*Lentinus edodes*（Berk.）Sing.的子实体。

【采收加工或制法】

春、秋、冬季均可采收，采得后除去泥沙杂质，晒干或焙干，备用。

【性味】味甘，性平，无毒。

【归经】入肝、胃经。

【功用】

扶正补虚，健脾开胃，祛风托毒，破血止遗。适宜于神疲力乏，纳食不馨，麻疹不透，小便失禁等病症者食用。

【服食方法】

可用于煲汤、炒食、煮粥等。

【食宜食忌】

脾胃寒湿气滞者禁食。

【储藏】

放阴凉、干燥处保存。

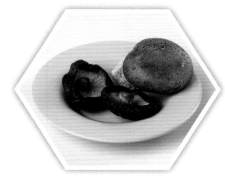

Xiang Gu

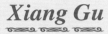

Shiitake Mushroom

【Origin】

It is the sporocarp of *Lentinus edodes*(Berk.)Sing. of *Lentinus* plant of family Tricholomataceae.

【Collection / Processing】

It can be collected in spring, autumn and winter. Remove the impurities such as the silts. Then dry the mushroom in the sun or by the fire for use.

【Flavor / Properties】 Sweet in flavor, moderate in nature and non-toxic.

【Meridian Tropism】 Liver and Stomach.

【Functions and Indications】

Reinforce the healthy *qi* and tonify deficiency, invigorate spleen and stimulate appetite, dispel wind and expel toxin, break blood stasis and restrain incontinence. Used for spiritlessness and fatigue, poor appetite, measles failing to let out, incontinence of urine, etc.

【Preparation / Consumption】

Cook soup, stir-fried or cook porridge.

【Cautions / Contraindications】

The one who has cold-damp and *qi* stagnation of spleen and stomach should not take it.

【Storage】

Preserved in cool and dry place.

银 耳
Yin Er

【基原或来源】

为真菌类银耳科银耳属植物银耳*Tremella fuciformis* Berk.的子实体。

【采收加工或制法】

当耳片开齐停止生长时，应及时采收，清水漂洗3次后，及时晒干或烘干。选材以耳花大而松散，耳肉肥厚，色呈白色或略带微黄，蒂头无黑斑者为佳。

【性味】味甘、淡，性平。

【归经】入肺、胃、肾经。

【功用】

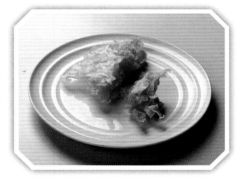

润肺养胃，化痰止咳，强心益智。适宜于肺胃阴虚，虚劳咳嗽，肺燥干咳，津少口渴，病后体虚，老年慢性支气管炎，肺结核，便秘者使用。

【服食方法】

可煮汤，做甜羹，煮粥，炒食，凉拌，或制作罐头等。

【食宜食忌】

肺胃阴虚所致口渴咽干、便秘者宜食；风寒咳嗽者及湿热酿痰致咳者慎食。煮熟的银耳存放过久后不宜再食用，因在细菌分解作用下，银耳中所含的较多的硝酸盐类会还原成亚硝酸盐，有致癌作用。

【储藏】

干品可放于阴凉、干燥、通风处保存，要注意防潮防蛀。

Yin Er

White Tremella

【Origin】
　　The fruiting body of *Tremella fuciformis* Berk. of *Tremella* genus in the family of Tremellaceae, Eumycophyta.

【Collection / Processing】
　　It should be harvested promptly when the leaves are fully blossomed and cease growing. After rinsed in water for 3 times, it should be sunned or baked to be dried promptly. Tips for purchase: it is advised to choose the one with big, loosening and fleshy leaves, with white or slightly yellowish color, and no dark spots in the end of pedicle.

【Flavor / Properties】 Sweet and bland in flavor, and neutral in nature.

【Meridian Tropism】 Lung, Stomach, and Kidney.

【Functions and Indications】
　　Moisturize the lung and nourish the stomach, resolve phlegm and stop coughing, strengthen the heart and boost the intelligence. Recommended for those with *yin* deficiency in the lung and the stomach, consumptive disease and cough, lung dryness and dry cough, thirst due to less body fluid, weakness after diseases, senile chronic bronchitis senile, pulmonary tuberculosis, or constipation.

【Preparation / Consumption】 It can be boiled, made into sweet thick soup, or porridge, and it can also be stir-fried, or cold blended, or made into canned foods.

【Cautions / Contraindications】
　　Highly recommended for those with thirst and dry pharynx due to *yin* deficiency in the lung and the stomach, or constipation. Use caution for those with cough due to wind-cold evil, or cough due to the phlegm caused by dampness-heat. The cooked white tremella should not be used after stored for a long time, because nitrates in white tremella will deoxidized into nitrite, which is carcinogenic, under the action of bacteria decomposition.

【Storage】
　　The dried one can be stored in cool, dry, and ventilated area, moisture and moth proofing.

马铃薯
Ma Ling Shu

【基原或来源】

为茄科茄属植物马铃薯*Solanum tuberosum* L.的块茎。

【采收加工或制法】

4～5月或9～10月挖取块茎，鲜用或晒干。

【性味】味甘，性平。

【归经】入脾、胃经。

【功用】

健脾和胃，降气通便，解毒消肿。适用于脾胃气虚，营养不良，嘈杂胃痛，大便秘结，疖腮痈肿，湿疹烫伤者使用。

【服食方法】

煮、炒，煎炸，焯后凉拌，加工成淀粉或粉丝等食用。

【食宜食忌】

脾胃虚寒易腹泻者宜少食。

【储藏】

放阴凉干燥处保存。

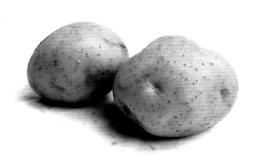

Ma Ling Shu

Potato

【Origin】

The tuber of *Solanum tuberosum* L.of *Solanum* genus in the family of Solanaceae.

【Collection / Processing】

Collect the tuber during April to May or September to October. Use fresh or after been dried.

【Flavor / Properties】 Sweet in flavor and moderate in nature.

【Meridian Tropism】 Spleen and Stomach.

【Functions and Indications】

Invigorate spleen and harmonize stomach, direct *qi* downward and frees the stool, remove toxin and disperse swelling. Recommended for those with deficiency of spleen-stomach *qi*, malnutrition, epigastric upset and stomachache, constipation, mumps and swelling, eczema and scald.

【Preparation / Consumption】

Boiled, stir-fried, deep-fried, mixed with other foods after blanched, made into starch or vermicelli.

【Cautions / Contraindications】

Frequent use and consumption of high quantities is not recommended for those with deficiency-cold of spleen and stomach or who are easy to have diarrhea.

【Storage】

Preserved in shady and dry place.

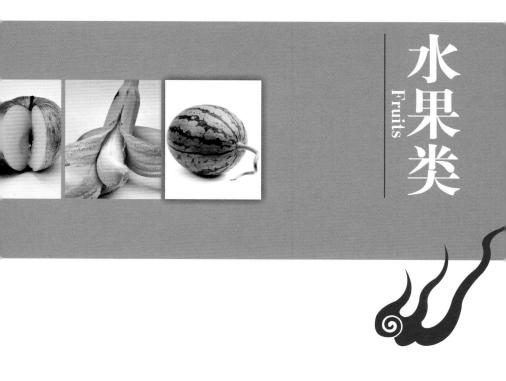

水果类
Fruits

西 瓜
Xi Gua

【基原或来源】

　　为葫芦科植物西瓜*Citrullus lanatus* (Thunb.) Matsum. et Nakai的果瓤。

【采收加工或制法】

　　夏季采摘。

【性味】味甘，性寒。

【归经】入心、胃、膀胱经。

【功用】

　　清热解暑，生津止渴，除烦利尿。适宜于暑热烦渴，热盛津伤，小便不利、水肿，喉痹口疮者食用。

【食宜食忌】

　　脾胃虚寒、泄泻、女子经期勿食或慎食。

【储藏】

　　放阴凉处保存。

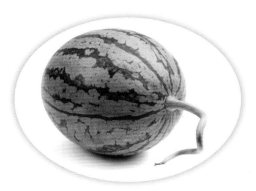

Xi Gua

Watermelon

【Origin】
　The pulp of *Citrullus lanatus* (Thunb.) Matsum. et Nakai in the family of Cucurbitaceae.

【Collection / Processing】
　Pick in summer.

【Flavor / Properties】 Sweet in flavor, cold in nature.

【Meridian Tropism】 Heart, Stomach and Bladder.

【Functions and Indications】
　Clear summer-heat, promote the production of saliva to slake thirst, remove restlessness and promote urination. Polydipsia, summer-heat, exuberant heat with damaging saliva difficult urination, edema, pharyngitis and aphtha.

【Cautions / Contraindications】
　Those with deficiency-cold of spleen and stomach, diarrhea and woman in menstrual period must not or should be cautious to take it.

【Storage】
　It should be preserved in shady and cool place.

苹 果
Ping Guo

【基原或来源】

　　为蔷薇科植物苹果*Malus pumila* Mill.的果实。

【采收加工或制法】

　　夏秋季采摘成熟果实。

【性味】味甘、酸，性凉，无毒。

【归经】入肺、胃经。

【功用】

　　生津润肺，解暑除烦，开胃醒酒。用于津少口渴，脾虚泄泻，食后腹胀，饮酒过度。

【服食方法】

　　鲜食，煮食，捣汁或熬膏食。

【食宜食忌】

　　胃寒者慎食，患有糖尿病者不宜多食。

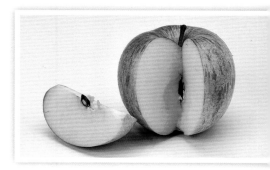

【储藏】

　　置阴凉处保存。

Ping Guo

Apple

【Origin】

It is the fruit of *Malus pumila* Mill. of family Rosaceae.

【Collection / Processing】

Collect the ripe fruit in summer or autumn.

【Flavor / Properties】 Sweet and sour in flavor, cool in nature and non-toxic.

【Meridian Tropism】 Lung and Stomach.

【Functions and Indications】

Generate fluid and moisten lung, clear summer heat and relieve vexation, stimulate appetite and sober up. Used for thirst due to lack of fluid, diarrhea due to spleen deficiency, abdominal distention after eating, over drinking.

【Preparation / Consumption】

Take the fruit fresh, cook it, squeeze juice or make paste.

【Cautions / Contraindications】

The one who has stomach cold should take it with caution, and the diabetic should not take it too much.

【Storage】

Preserved in cool place.

梨
Li

【基原或来源】

为蔷薇科植物白梨*Pyrus bretschneideri* Rehd、沙梨*Pyrus pyrifolia*（Burm.f.）Nakai、秋子梨*Pyrus ussuriensis* Maxim等栽培种的果实。

【采收加工或制法】

8～9月间果实成熟时采收。

【性味】味甘、微酸，性凉，无毒。

【归经】入肺、胃、心经。

【功用】

清心除烦，生津止渴，消痰醒酒，润肠通便。用于热病津伤，心烦口渴，痰热咳嗽，中风不语，失音咽干，便秘尿涩，疮毒酒毒。

【服食方法】

生食、捣汁、煎汤、蒸服、熬膏等。

【食宜食忌】

脾虚便溏、寒嗽及产妇忌食或慎食。

【储藏】

鲜品宜在阴凉、湿润、通风处保存。

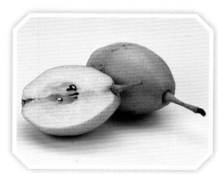

Li

Pear

【Origin】

The pears are the fruits of cultivated species of *Pyrus bretschneideri* Rehd, *Pyrus pyrifolia* (Burm.f.) Nakai and *Pyrus ussuriensis* Maxim of family Rosaceae.

【Collection / Processing】

Herborized during August and September when the fruits are ripe.

【Flavor / Properties】 Sweet and slight sour in flavor, cool in nature and non-toxic.

【Meridian Tropism】 Lung, Stomach and Heart.

【Functions and Indications】

Clear heart-fire to relieve dysphoria, generate body fluid to quench thirst, dissolve phlegm and dispel the effects of alcohol, moisten intestine to relieve constipation. Commonly used for vexation and thirst due to febrile disease that causes body fluid consumption, cough due to phlegm heat, aphasia from apoplexy, aphonia and dry throat, constipation and difficult urination, poisonous sores and alcoholism.

【Preparation / Consumption】

The pears can be taken in the fresh form, or be used to squeeze juice, cook soup, be stewed or make paste, etc.

【Contraindications / Cautions】

The one who has diarrhea due to spleen deficiency, cold cough and the puerpera should take it with caution or not take it.

【Storage】

The fresh fruits should preserved in cool, moist and well-ventilated place.

桃 子
Tao Zi

【基原或来源】

为蔷薇科植物桃*Amygdalus persica* L.或山桃*A. davidiana* (Carr.)C.de Vos ex Henry.的果实。

【采收加工或制法】

6～7月果实成熟时采摘。

【性味】味甘、酸，性温。无毒。

【归经】入肝、肺、大肠经。

【功用】

生津润肠，活血消积。用于津少口渴，咳逆上气，肠燥便秘，积聚闭经。

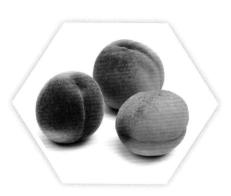

【服食方法】

鲜食，作脯食，制酱、榨汁或制桃罐头。

【食宜食忌】

不宜多食。

【储藏】

鲜桃放阴凉处保存。

Tao Zi

Peach

【Origin】
The fruit of *Amygdalus persica* L. or *A. davidiana* (Carr.) C.de Vos ex Henry. in the Family of Rosaceae.

【Collection / Processing】
Harvest the ripe fruits in June and July.

【Flavor / Properties】 Sweet and sour in flavor, warm in nature, and nontoxic.

【Meridian Tropism】 Liver, Lung, and Large Intestine.

【Functions and Indications】
Engender the fluids and moisten the intestines, promote blood circulation to remove stagnation. Used for thirst due to inadequate fluids, cough with dyspnea, dryness of the intestine and constipation, accumulation and amenorrhea.

【Preparation / Consumption】
It can be eaten fresh, made into preserved fruit, jelly and juice, or canned.

【Cautions / Contraindications】
Consumption of high quantities is not recommended.

【Storage】
The fresh should be preserved in shady place.

杏 子
Xing Zi

【基原或来源】

　　为蔷薇科植物杏*Armeniaca vulgaris* Lam.或山杏*Armeniaca sibirica* Lam.等的果实。

【采收加工或制法】

　　夏季果熟时采收。

【性味】味酸、甘，性温。

【归经】入肺、心经。

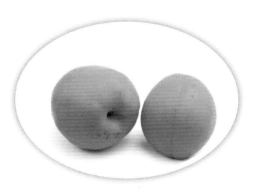

【功用】

　　润肺生津，止咳定喘，解毒。适宜于肺燥咳嗽，心烦口渴者食用。

【服食方法】

　　鲜食，煮粥，制杏干、杏脯。

【食宜食忌】

　　不宜多食；患皮肤痒疹者慎食。

【储藏】

　　放阴凉干燥处保存。

Xing Zi

Apricot

【Origin】
The fruit of *Armeniaca vulgaris* Lam. or *Armeniaca sibirica* Lam. in the family of Rosaceae.

【Collection / Processing】
Pick when the fruit is mature in summer.

【Flavor / Properties】 Sour and sweet in flavor, warm in nature.

【Meridian Tropism】 Lung and Heart.

【Functions and Indications】
Promote production of body fluid and moisten lung, relieve cough, relieve asthma, and detoxicate. Lung dryness, cough, and polydipsia.

【Preparation / Consumption】
It can be taken uncooked, cooked in congee, or processed into dried or preserved apricot.

【Cautions / Contraindications】
It should not be taken much; those with skin prurigo should be cautious to take it.

【Storage】
It should be preserved in shady, cool and dry place.

香 蕉
Xiang Jiao

【基原或来源】

为芭蕉科植物甘蕉*Musa paradisiaca* L. var. *sapientum* (L.) O. Kuntze、香蕉 *Musa nana* Lour.的果实。

【采收加工或制法】

秋季果实将成熟时采收。

【性味】味甘，性寒。

【归经】入肺、胃、大肠经。

【功用】

清热解毒，润肺通便。用于热病烦渴，肺燥咳嗽，便秘痔疮。

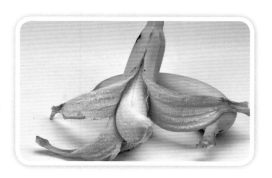

【服食方法】

鲜食、炖熟食、蜜渍、制果干食。

【食宜食忌】

女子经期、脾胃虚寒便溏泄泻者慎食。

【储藏】

放凉爽通风处保存。

Xiang Jiao

Banana

【Origin】
The fruit of *Musa paradisiaca* L. var. *sapientum* (L.) O. Kuntze or *Musa nana* Lour. in the family of Musaceae.

【Collection / Processing】
Pick when the fruit is to be mature in autumn.

【Flavor / Properties】 Sweet in flavor, cold in nature.

【Meridian Tropism】 Lung, Stomach and Large Intestine.

【Functions and Indications】
Clear heat, detoxicate, moisten lung and relax bowels. Pyreticosis and polydipsia, lung dryness, cough, constipation and haemorrhoid.

【Preparation / Consumption】
It can be taken uncooked, stewed, candied and processed into dry fruit.

【Cautions / Contraindications】
Those with deficiency-cold of spleen and stomach, loose stool or diarrhea and woman in menstrual period should be cautious to take it.

【Storage】
It should be preserved in cool and ventilate place.

葡 萄
Pu Tao

【基原或来源】

为葡萄科植物葡萄*Vitis vinifera* L.的果实。

【采收加工或制法】

夏末秋初果熟时采收。

【性味】味甘、酸，性平。无毒。

【归经】入肺、脾、肾经。

【功用】

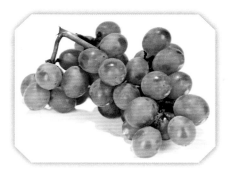

补气血，益肝肾，生津液，强筋骨，利小便。适用于气血虚弱，肺虚咳嗽，心悸盗汗，烦渴，风湿痹病，淋证浮肿，麻疹不透者使用。

【服食方法】

生食、捣汁、熬膏、煮粥、浸酒食或浸酒后外用。

【食宜食忌】

阴虚内热、实热内盛者慎食，不宜多食。

【储藏】

鲜品放阴凉干燥处保存，干品置干燥处容器内，防热、防潮、防蛀。

Pu Tao

Grape

【Origin】
The fruit of *Vitis vinifera* L. in the *family* of Vitaceae.

【Collection / Processing】
Harvested in the late summer or the early autumn when it is ripe.

【Flavor / Properties】 Sweet and acid in flavor, moderate in nature, and nontoxic.

【Meridian Tropism】 Lung, Spleen, and Kidney.

【Functions and Indications】
Tonify *qi* and blood, replenish the liver and kidney, engender the body fluids, strengthen bones and muscles, and promote urination. Recommended for those with weakness of *qi* and blood , cough due to deficiency of the lung, night sweat due to palpitations, polydipsia, rheumatic arthralgia, swelling due to stranguria, or measles without adequate eruption.

【Preparation / Consumption】
It can be eaten raw, or after be made into juice, boiled to a paste, boiled into porridge, or steeped in wine. It can also be used externally after be steeped in wine.

【Cautions / Contraindications】
Use caution for those with *yin* deficiency with internal heat, or severe intrinsic sthenic heat. Consumption of high quantities is not recommended.

【Storage】
The fresh should be preserved in shady and dry place, and the dried should be preserved in dry containers. Heat, moisture, and moth should be prevented.

菠 萝
Bo Luo

【基原或来源】

为凤梨科凤梨属植物菠萝*Ananas comosre* (L.) Merr.的果实。

【采收加工或制法】

春果4~5月成熟后采收；夏果6~7月采收；秋果10~11月采收；冬果12月至翌年1月采收。以果形端正饱满，果皮淡黄富有光泽，软硬适中，具芳香气味者为佳。

【性味】味甘、酸、微涩，性平。

【归经】入肺、胃经。

【功用】

清暑止渴，开胃消食。适宜于中暑，烦热不安，口干咽燥，食欲不振，消化不良，肺胃阴虚，腹泻，脘腹痞满，小便不利，支气管炎者使用。

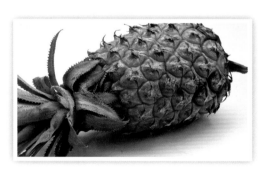

【服食方法】

可生食，榨汁，凉拌，炒食，做汤，做膏，制作罐头、蜜饯、果酱、果酒、果汁，提制柠檬酸等。食用前宜用淡盐水浸泡1小时左右，可破坏菠萝蛋白酶，防止过敏。

【食宜食忌】

身热烦躁者、消化不良者宜食；过敏体质者、低血压、内脏下垂者慎食。

【储藏】

未削皮者可放于阴凉、通风处保存；已削皮者可用保鲜膜封好放冰箱暂存。

Bo Luo

Pineapple

【Origin】

The fruit of *Ananas comosus* (L.) Merr. of *Ananas* genus in the family of Bromeliaceae.

【Collection / Processing】

The spring fruit can be collected during April to May, the summer fruit during June to July, the autumn fruit during October to November, and the winter fruit during December to January of the next year. Tips for purchase: it is advised to choose the one with full shape, yellowish and shiny peel, moderate hardness, and with fragrant smell.

【Flavor / Properties】 Sweet, sour and slightly pungent in flavor, neutral in nature.

【Meridian Tropism】 Lung and Stomach.

【Functions and Indications】

Clear summer-heat and quench thirst, increase appetite and promote digestion. Recommended for those with heatstroke, feverish dysphoria, dry mouth and throat, poor appetite, dyspepsia, deficiency of lung-stomach *yin*, diarrhea, chest-abdomen fullness, difficulty in micturition, or bronchitis.

【Preparation / Consumption】

It can be eaten directly, or made into juice, salad, soup, paste, it can also be stir-fried, made into canned goods, conserves, fruit jam, fruit wine, juice, or used to extract citric acid. It should be better to be soaked in salt water for one hour before consumption, for bromelain can be broken down after that to prevent allergy.

【Cautions / Contraindications】

Highly recommended for those with feverish dysphoria or dyspepsia. Use caution for those with allergic constitution, hypotension, or visceroptosis.

【Storage】

The unpeeled one can be stored in shady and ventilated area, and the peeled one can be sealed up with freshness-keeping plastic film to be temporarily kept in refrigerator.

草 莓
Cao Mei

【基原或来源】

为蔷薇科草莓属植物草莓*Fragaria ananassa* Duch.的果实。

【采收加工或制法】

夏季6～7月采摘。选购时以果体大小适中而完整、果皮鲜红光亮、有细微茸毛者为佳。

【性味】味甘、酸，性凉。

【归经】入肺、脾、胃经。

【功用】

清热生津，润肺止咳，开胃消食。适宜于中暑，肺胃阴虚，口干咽燥，风热咳嗽，食欲不振，小便短赤，便秘，贫血，疮疖，癌症者使用。

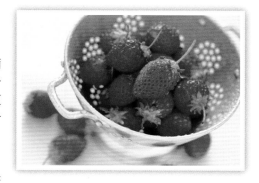

【服食方法】

可生吃，榨汁，凉拌，制作果酱、果酒、果汁、果冻、罐头等。

【食宜食忌】

肺寒痰白而多者、脾胃虚寒易泄泻者慎食；草莓中含草酸钙较多，故结石患者不宜多食。

【储藏】

不要清洗，可直接将带蒂的草莓用保鲜膜封好，放入冰箱冷藏。

Cao Mei

Strawberry

【Origin】
It is the fruit of *Fragaria ananassa* Duch. of family Rosaceae.

【Collection / Processing】
Collect the fruit during June and July in summer. Choose the fruit in proper size with bright red pericarp and fine fuzzes.

【Flavor / Properties】 Sweet and sour in flavor, cool in nature.

【Meridian Tropism】 Lung, Spleen and Stomach.

【Functions and Indications】
Clear heat and generate fluid, moisten lung and stop cough, promote appetite and digestion. Used for heatstroke, deficiency of lung-stomach *yin*, dry mouth and throat, cough due to wind-heat, poor appetite, short and dark urine, constipation, anemia, sores and furuncles, cancer, etc.

【Preparation / Consumption】
Take the fresh fruit, squeeze juice, mix with sauce or make jam, wine, juice, jelly and tins.

【Cautions / Contraindications】
The one who has much white sputum due to lung cold or diarrhea due to spleen and stomach deficiency-cold should take the fruit with caution. Besides, the patient with calculus should not take the fruit too much because there is much calcium oxalate in strawberry.

【Storage】
The fresh strawberry with pedicle can be sealed with preservative film without cleaning and refrigerated in a freezer.

大 枣
Da Zao

【基原或来源】

为鼠李科植物枣 *Ziziphus jujuba* Mill. 的成熟果实。

【采收加工或制法】

秋季果实成熟时采收。

【性味】 味甘，性温，无毒。

【归经】 入心、脾、胃经。

【功用】

补脾益胃，养血安神，缓和药性。用于脾虚泄泻，体倦乏力，纳食量少，心悸怔忡，失眠盗汗，妇人脏躁。

【服食方法】

鲜食、煮粥、蒸熟食。

【食宜食忌】

湿痰痰热、积滞中满、牙病疼痛者忌食。

【储藏】

置干燥处，防蛀。

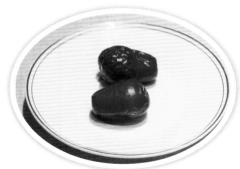

Da Zao

Chinese Date

【Origin】
It is the ripe fruit of *Ziziphus jujuba* Mill. of family Rhamnaceae.

【Collection / Processing】
Herborized when the fruits are ripe in autumn.

【Flavor / Properties】 Sweet in flavor, warm in nature, and non-toxic.

【Meridian Tropism】 Heart, Spleen, and Stomach.

【Functions and Indications】
Tonify spleen and replenish stomach, nourish blood and tranquilize mind, and moderate drug nature. Commonly used for diarrhea due to insufficiency of the spleen, weary and acratia, severe palpitation, insomnia and night sweat, and hysteria of woman.

【Preparation / Consumption】
Can be taken when fresh, cooked congee, or taken after steamed.

【Contraindications / Cautions】
It is contraindicated for people with damp-phlegm, dyspeptic disease and abdominal flatulence, and toothache.

【Storage】
It should be stored in dry and moth proofing places.

橘
Ju

【基原或来源】

为芸香科植物橘*Citrus reticulata* Blanco.及其栽培变种的成熟果实。

【采收加工或制法】

10～12月果实成熟时采摘。

【性味】味甘、酸，性凉，无毒。

【归经】入肺、心、胃经。

【功用】

润肺止渴，理气宽胸，解酒和胃。适宜于干咳无痰，烦热口渴，胸膈结气，伤酒呃逆者食用。

【服食方法】

鲜食、制作罐头、入药膳等。

【食宜食忌】

不宜多食，风寒咳嗽及痰湿盛者忌食。

【储藏】

放阴凉干燥处或冷藏保存。

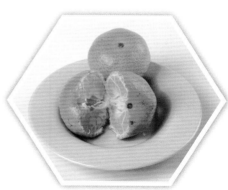

Ju

Tangerine

【Origin】

It is the ripe fruit of *Citrus reticulata* Blanco. and its varietal plant of family Rutaceae.

【Collection / Processing】

Collect the ripe fruits during October and December.

【Flavor / Properties】 Sweet and sour in flavor, cool in nature and non-toxic.

【Meridian Tropism】 Lung, Heart and Stomach.

【Functions and Indications】

Moisten lung and quench thirst, regulate *qi* and relieve chest distress, sober up and harmonize stomach. Used for dry cough without sputum, vexation and fever, thirst, qi stagnation in chest and diaphragm, sick due to over drinking, hiccup, etc.

【Preparation / Consumption】

Take the fresh fruit, make cans or medicated diet.

【Cautions / Contraindications】

It should not be taken too much and it is forbidden for the one who has cough due to wind-cold and excessive sputum and dampness.

【Storage】

Preserved in cool and dry place or refrigerated.

金 橘
Jin Ju

【基原或来源】

为芸香科植物金橘*Fortunella margarita* (Lour.) Swingle.和金弹*Fortunella crassifolia* Swingle.等的果实。

【采收加工或制法】

果实成熟时采摘。

【性味】味辛、甘，性温。

【归经】入肝、肺、胃经。

【功用】

理气解郁，消食化痰，醒酒止渴。适宜于胸闷气滞，咳嗽痰多，脘腹痞胀，纳呆口臭，伤酒口渴者食用。

【服食方法】

鲜食；或捣汁饮，或泡茶。

【食宜食忌】

不宜与牛奶同食，糖尿病患者忌用。

【储藏】

放阴凉干燥处保存。

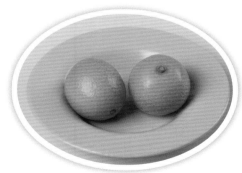

Jin Ju

Kumquat

【Origin】
It is the fruit of *Fortunella margarita* (Lour.) Swingle. and *Fortunella crassifolia* Swingle. of family Rutaceae.

【Collection / Processing】
Collect the ripe fruits.

【Flavor / Properties】 Pungent and sweet in flavor, warm in nature.

【Meridian Tropism】 Liver, Lung and Stomach.

【Functions and Indications】
Regulate *qi* and relieve depression, promote digestion and resolve sputum, sober up and quench thirst. Used for chest distress and *qi* stagnation, cough with much sputum, abdominal distention, poor appetite and halitosis, sick due to over drinking, thirst, etc.

【Preparation / Consumption】
Take the fresh fruit, squeeze juice, or make tea.

【Cautions / Contraindications】
It should not be taken with milk and it is forbidden for the diabetic.

【Storage】
Preserved in cool and dry place.

荔 枝
Li Zhi

【基原或来源】

为无患子科荔枝属植物荔枝*Litchi chinensis* Sonn.的果实。

【采收加工或制法】

6~7月果实成熟时采集，鲜食或晒干。

【性味】味甘、酸，性温，无毒。

【归经】入脾、肝经。

【功用】

养血生津，健脾行气，消肿止痛。用于病后体虚，津伤烦渴，脾虚泄泻，胃痛呃逆，牙疼口臭，瘰疬疔肿。

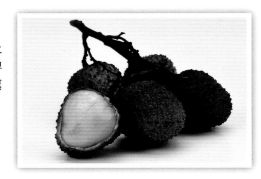

【服食方法】

鲜食、煎汤或浸酒。

【食宜食忌】

阴虚火旺者慎食。

【储藏】

鲜果低温保存，干品密封贮藏。

Li Zhi

Litchi Chinensis

【Origin】

It is the fruit of *Litchi chinensis* Sonn. of family Sapindaceae.

【Collection / Processing】

Herborized during June and July when the fruit is ripe. Take the fruit when it is fresh or after being dried in the sun.

【Flavor / Properties】 Sweet and sour in flavor, warm in nature and non-toxic.

【Meridian Tropism】 Spleen and Liver.

【Functions and Indications】

Nourish blood and generate body fluid, invigorate spleen and promote *qi* circulation, reduce swelling and relieve pain. Commonly used for the sick, polydipsia due to body fluid consumption, diarrhea due to spleen deficiency, stomachache and hiccup, toothache and halitosis, scrofula and furuncles, etc.

【Preparation / Consumption】

Can be taken in the fresh form, be used to cook soup or soak in the wine.

【Contraindications / Cautions】

The one who has *yin* deficiency with effulgent fire should take it with caution.

【Storage】

The fresh fruit should be stored in low temperature while the dried form should be preserved in airtight container.

杧 果
Mang Guo

【基原或来源】

为漆树科杧果属植物杧果*Mangifera indica* L.的果实。

【采收加工或制法】

夏、秋季节采摘成熟果实，鲜用或晒干备用。以果大饱满，表皮光滑、颜色均匀，富含果汁者为佳。

【性味】 味酸、甘，性平。无毒。

【归经】 入肝、肺、脾、胃经。

【功用】

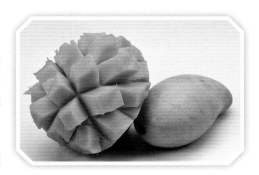

益胃止呕，生津止渴，止咳利尿。适宜于胃热口渴，眩晕症，高血压头晕，美尼尔综合征，恶心欲吐，小便不利，咳嗽气喘者使用。

【服食方法】

可鲜食，蜜饯，亦可作果干、罐头、果酒等，未成熟之果实可制果酱、果醋饮品或腌制。

【食宜食忌】

口干，眩晕，小便不利，咳喘者尤宜食用。糖尿病患者不宜食。过敏体质或皮肤易过敏者食用时宜慎。

【储藏】

鲜果置阴凉通风处可保存1周左右。或晒干后，置于密封干燥容器内，防潮、防霉。

Mang Guo

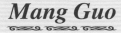

Mango

【Origin】
The fruit of *Mangifera indica* L. of *Mangifera* genus in the family of Anacardiaceae.

【Collection / Processing】
Collect the ripe fruits in summer or autumn, use fresh or get them dried. Tips for purchase: it is advised to choose the one with full shape and big size, glossy pericarp, uniform color, and rich juice.

【Flavor / Properties】 Sour and sweet in flavor, neutral in nature, and non-toxic.

【Meridian Tropism】 Liver, Lung, Spleen and Stomach.

【Functions and Indications】
Nourish the stomach and stop vomit, promote the production of body fluid to quench thirst, relieve cough and induce diuresis. Recommended for those with thirst due to stomach heat, vertigo, dizziness due to hypertension, Meniere's syndrome, nausea and vomit, difficulty in micturition, or cough with asthma.

【Preparation / Consumption】
It can be used fresh, or made into conserves, dried fruits, canned goods, or fruit wine. The green fruits can be used to make fruit jam or fruit vinegar, or to be pickled.

【Cautions / Contraindications】
Highly recommended for those with thirst, dizziness, difficulty in micturition, or cough with asthma. Not recommended for those with diabetes. Be caution for those with allergic constitution or skin allergy.

【Storage】
The fresh fruit can be stored in shady and ventilated place for about one week. It can also be dried and sealed up in dry containers for storage, moisture and mould proofing.

龙眼肉
Long Yan Rou

【基原或来源】

　　为无患子科植物龙眼 *Euphoria longan*（Lour）．Steud 的假种皮。

【采收加工或制法】

　　7～10月果实成熟时采摘。

【性味】味甘，性温，无毒。

【归经】入心、脾经。

【功用】

　　补益心脾，养血安神。用于心脾两虚引起的心悸怔忡，失眠健忘，头昏眼花，面色萎黄，月经不调等。

【服食方法】

　　鲜食、泡茶、煮粥、熬膏、制果羹、浸酒后食。

【食宜食忌】

　　外感表证、内有痰火及湿滞停饮者忌服。

【储藏】

　　干品置通风干燥处，防潮，防蛀。

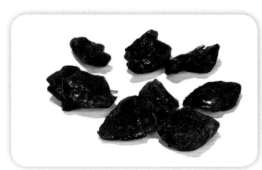

Long Yan Rou

Arillus Longanae

【Origin】
The aril of *Euphoria longan* (Lour). Steud in the family of Sapindaceae.

【Collection / Processing】
Collect the ripe fruits during July to October.

【Flavor / Properties】 Sweet in flavor, warm in nature, and nontoxic.

【Meridian Tropism】 Heart and Spleen.

【Functions and Indications】
Tonify heart and spleen, nourish blood and tranquilize mind. It can be used for severe palpitation caused by heart and spleen deficiency, insomnia and forgetfulness, dizziness, etiolated face, or abnormal menstrual.

【Preparation / Consumption】
Fresh consumption, or use after brewed as tea, boiled into porridge, made into paste, fruit soup, or macerated in wine.

【Cautions / Contraindications】
Contraindicated for those with exterior pattern of external contraction, and phlegm-fire, damp stagnancy in the interior.

【Storage】
Store the dried one in aired, dried, moisture and moth proofing area.

枇 杷
Pi Pa

【基原或来源】

为蔷薇科植物枇杷*Eriobotrya japonica*（Thunb.）Lindl. (*Mespilus japonica* Thunb.)的果实。

【采收加工或制法】

果实成熟时分次采摘。

【性味】味甘、酸，性凉。

【归经】入脾、肺、肝经。

【功用】

清热止渴，润肺下气，化痰止咳，和胃止呕。适宜于肺热咳嗽，烦渴，呕逆者食用。

【服食方法】

鲜食，煮粥，制膏，制枇杷罐头，酿酒等。

【食宜食忌】

脾胃虚寒者忌用。

【储藏】

放阴凉处保存，或制成蜜饯久藏。

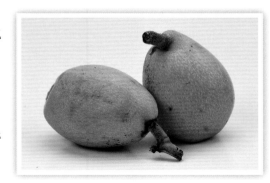

Pi Pa

Loquat

【Origin】

It is the fruit of *Eriobotrya japonica* (Thunb.) Lindl. (Mespilus japonica Thunb.) of family Rosaceae.

【Collection / Processing】

Collect the ripe fruits separately.

【Flavor / Properties】 Sweet and sour in flavor, cool in nature.

【Meridian Tropism】 Spleen, Lung and Liver.

【Functions and Indications】

Clear heat to quench thirst, moisten lung and descend *qi*, resolve phlegm and relieve cough, harmonize stomach to prevent vomit. Used for cough due to lung heat, vexation and thirst, vomit.

【Preparation / Consumption】

Take the fresh fruit, cook porridge, make paste, fruit can or wine, etc.

【Cautions / Contraindications】

The one who has deficiency-cold of spleen and stomach should not take it.

【Storage】

Preserved in cool place or processed as glace fruit for long time preservation.

柿
Shi

【基原或来源】

为柿树科植物柿*Diospyros kaki* Thunb.的果实。

【采收加工或制法】

霜降至立冬间采摘，经脱涩红熟后鲜食。

【性味】 味甘、涩，性凉。无毒。

【归经】 入心、肺、大肠经。

【功用】

清热生津，润肺止咳，涩肠止血。适宜于肺燥咳嗽，反胃呕吐，吐血咯血，血淋痢疾，痔漏下血者食之。

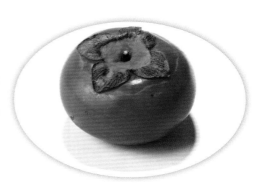

【服食方法】

鲜食、制柿饼或煮粥食。

【食宜食忌】

凡脾胃虚寒，痰湿内盛，外感咳嗽，脾虚泄泻及空腹均不宜食。

【储藏】

鲜柿阴凉处保存，干柿密封贮藏。

Shi

Persimmon

【Origin】

The fruit of *Diospyros kaki* Thunb. in the Family of Ebenaceae.

【Collection / Processing】

Collected from first frost to the beginning of winter, and it should be eaten fresh after the astringent flavor disappears and the color turns into red.

【Flavor / Properties】 Sweet and astringent in flavor, cool in nature, and nontoxic.

【Meridian Tropism】 Heart, Lung and Large Intestine.

【Functions and Indications】

Remove heat and promote fluid production, moisten lung to arrest cough, astringe intestines and stop bleeding. Recommended for those with cough of lung dryness, regurgitation and vomiting, blood-spitting and hemoptysis, bloody stranguria and dysentery, or anus fistula.

【Preparation / Consumption】

It should be eaten when fresh, made into persimmon cake, or boiled into porridge.

【Cautions / Contraindications】

Those with deficiency-cold of spleen and stomach, phlegm-damp of exuberant internal, externally contracted cough, or spleen-asthenic diarrhea, and one on an empty stomach should avoid in consumption.

【Storage】

Preserve the fresh in shady place, and the dried by air-proof preservation.

无花果
Wu Hua Guo

【基原或来源】

为桑科植物无花果*Ficus carica* L.的果实。

【采收加工或制法】

秋季果实成熟时采收。洗净鲜用，或晒干用。

【性味】 味甘，性凉。无毒

【归经】 入肺、脾、大肠经。

【功用】

清热生津，润肺止咳，健脾开胃，解毒消肿。用于咽喉肿痛，燥咳声嘶，乳汁不足，泄泻痢疾，便秘痔疮，痈疮疥癣。

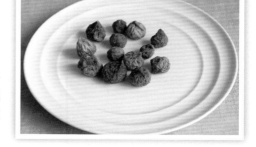

【服食方法】

鲜食，或制成果脯、果酱、饮料、罐头或用于烹饪菜肴。

【储藏】

鲜食，干果贮藏干燥处，防霉蛀。

Wu Hua Guo

Ficus Carica

【Origin】

The fruit of F*icus carica* L., plant in the family of Moraceae.

【Collection / Processing】

Pick when the fruit is mature in autumn, and wash for fresh use or dry in the sun.

【Flavor / Properties】 Sweet in flavor, cool in nature, and non-toxic.

【Meridian Tropism】 Lung, Spleen and Large Intestine.

【Functions and Indications】

Clear heat and promote fluid production, moisten lungs and relieve cough, improve spleen and stimulate appetite, detoxicate and reduce swelling. Sore throat, dry cough and hoarseness, hypogalactia, diarrhea and dysentery, constipation and hemorrhoid, abscess and scabies.

【Preparation / Consumption】

It can be taken fresh, processed into preserved fruit, jam, beverage and tin, or used for cooking.

【Storage】

It should be taken fresh, and dry fruit should be put in dry place, without damaged by mould.

甘 蔗
Gan Zhe

【基原或来源】

为禾本科植物甘蔗*Saccharum sinensis* Roxb.的茎秆。

【采收加工或制法】

秋后采收，砍取地上部分，去皮用。

【性味】味甘，性寒，无毒。

【归经】入肺、胃经。

【功用】

清热生津，润肺止咳，和中下气，解毒通便。治热病津伤，心烦口渴，肺燥咳嗽，咽喉肿痛，反胃呕吐，大便燥结，酒毒疮痈。

【服食方法】

嚼汁，或榨汁饮。外用捣敷。

【食宜食忌】

脾胃虚寒泄泻者慎食。

【储藏】

放阴暗不通风处，保持水分。

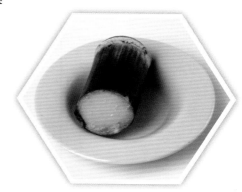

Gan Zhe

Sugarcane

【Origin】

It is the stalk of *Saccharum sinensis* Roxb. of family Poaceae.

【Collection / Processing】

Collect the cane in late autumn, cut the aboveground part and remove the peel.

【Flavor / Properties】 Sweet in flavor, cold in nature and non-toxic.

【Meridian Tropism】 Lung and Stomach.

【Functions and Indications】

Clear heat and promote fluid production, moisten lung to relieve cough, harmonize middle energizer and make the converse *qi* downward, detoxicate and relax the bowels. Used for body fluid consumption due to febrile disease, vexation and thirst, cough due to lung dryness, sore throat, regurgitation and vomit, dry stool, alcoholism and carbuncles.

【Preparation / Consumption】

Chew the juice or squeeze juice. Pound for external use.

【Cautions / Contraindications】

The one who has diarrhea due to deficiency-cold of spleen and stomach should take it with caution.

【Storage】

Preserved in shady and unventilated place to keep its moisture.

猕猴桃
Mi Hou Tao

【基原或来源】

为猕猴桃科植物猕猴桃*Actinidia chinensis* Planch.的果实。

【采收加工或制法】

夏末秋初采摘成熟果实，鲜食或晒干用。

【性味】 味甘、酸，性寒。

【归经】 入肾、胃经。

【功用】

调中下气，生津润燥，解热除烦，利尿通淋。适用于反胃呕吐，消渴烦热，黄疸石淋，便秘痔疮者使用。

【服食方法】

生食，做蜜饯，或榨汁饮。

【食宜食忌】

脾胃虚寒者慎食。

【储藏】

鲜品放阴凉干燥处保存，干品密封保存。

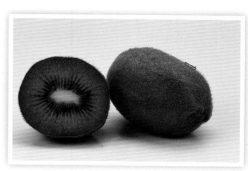

Mi Hou Tao

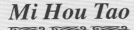

Kiwi Fruit

【Origin】
It is the fruit of *Actinidia chinensis* Planch. of family Actinidiaceae.

【Collection / Processing】
Collect the ripe fruit in late summer and early autumn, take the fresh fruit or dry the fruit in sun.

【Flavor / Properties】 Sweet and sour in flavor, cold in nature,

【Meridian Tropism】 Kidney and Stomach.

【Functions and Indications】
Regulate middle energizer and descend qi, generate fluid to moisten dryness, allay fever and relieve vexation, promote urination and relieve stranguria. Used for nausea and vomit, diabetes and vexation, jaundice and urolithiasis, constipation and hemorrhoids.

【Preparation / Consumption】
Take the raw fruit, make succade or squeeze juice.

【Cautions / Contraindications】
The one who has deficient-cold of spleen and stomach should take it with caution.

【Storage】
The fresh fruit should be preserved in cool and dry place and dried fruit should be preserved air-tightly.

荸 荠
Bi Qi

【基原或来源】

为莎草科植物荸荠*Heleocharis dulcis*（Burm.f.）Trin.ex Henschel的球茎。

【采收加工或制法】

10～12月挖取，洗净，风干或鲜用。

【性味】味甘，性寒，无毒。

【归经】入肺、胃经。

【功用】

清热化痰，生津止渴，开胃消食。适用于痰热咳嗽，热病口渴，咽喉肿痛，食积痢疾，黄疸热淋，目赤肿痛，便血崩漏者食用。

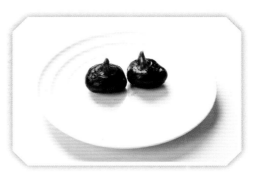

【服食方法】

生食、煮食、拌、炒、烧、煨、炸食，或捣汁，或浸酒，或澄粉等。

【食宜食忌】

虚寒及血虚者慎食。

【储藏】

鲜品阴凉处保存，干品密封保存。

Bi Qi

Water Chestnut

【Origin】

The corm of *Heleocharis dulcis* (Burm.f.) Trin.ex Henschel in the family of Cyperaceae.

【Collection / Processing】

Harvested during October to December. After cleaned, it can be used fresh or after been dried.

【Flavor / Properties】 Sweet in flavor, cold in nature, and nontoxic.

【Meridian Tropism】 Lung and Stomach.

【Functions and Indications】

Clear heat and eliminate phlegm, promote the production of body fluid to quench thirst, increase appetite and promote digestion. Recommended for those with phlegm-heat cough, febrile disease and thirst, sore swollen throat, food accumulation and dysentery, jaundice and heat strangury, sore read swollen eyes, bloody stool and uterine bleeding.

【Preparation / Consumption】

It can be eaten raw or after being cooked, or used for salad, stir-fried, cooked, roasted, or deep-fried. It can also be grinded to make juice, steeped in wine, or made into non-glutinous flour.

【Cautions / Contraindications】

Use with caution for those with deficiency-cold and blood-deficiency.

【Storage】

Preserve the fresh in shady place, and the dry with airproof preservation.

山 楂
Shan Zha

【基原或来源】

为蔷薇科植物山里红*Crataegus pinnatifida* Bunge．var．*major* N．E．Br．或山楂*Crataegus pinnatifida* Bunge．的成熟果实。

【采收加工或制法】

秋季果实成熟时采收。

【性味】酸、甘，微温。

【归经】入脾、胃、肝经。

【功用】

消食化积，行气散瘀，降血脂。用于饮食积滞，脘腹胀满，嗳腐吞酸，泄泻痢疾，血瘀痛经，产后腹痛，恶露不尽，疝气腹痛，阴囊肿胀疼痛，高血脂及肥胖病症等。

【服食方法】

可鲜食，熬膏，煎汤，煮粥，泡茶，榨汁等。

【食宜食忌】

脾胃虚弱者慎服。

【储藏】

干品置通风干燥处，防蛀。

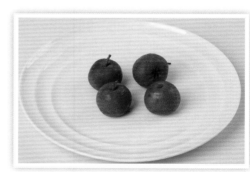

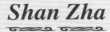

Shan Zha

Haw

【Origin】
It is the ripe fruit of *Crataegus pinnatifida* Bunge. var. *major* N.E. Br. or *Crataegus pinnatifida* Bunge. of family Rosaceae.

【Collection / Processing】
Herborized in autumn when the fruit is ripe.

【Flavor / Properties】 Sour and sweet in flavor, slightly warm.

【Meridian Tropism】 Spleen, Stomach and Liver.

【Functions and Indications】
Promote digestion and dissipate food stagnation, promote *qi* circulation and resolve blood stasis, lower the blood lipid. Commonly used for food stagnation, abdominal distention, belching and acid regurgitation, diarrhea due to dysentery, dysmenorrheal due to blood stasis, postpartum abdominal pain, endless lochia, abdominal pain due to hernia, swelling and pain of the scrotum, hyperlipidemia and obesity, etc.

【Preparation / Consumption】
Can be taken in the fresh form or be used to make paste, cook soup and porridge, make tea and squeeze juice, etc.

【Contraindications / Cautions】
The one who has weakened spleen and stomach function should take the material with caution.

【Storage】
The dried material should be preserved in aeration-drying place and prevented from the moth.

石 榴
Shi Liu

【基原或来源】

石榴科植物石榴 *Punica granatum* L.的果实。

【采收加工或制法】

9~10月果实成熟后采集，鲜食。

【性味】味酸，或甘、涩。性温。

【归经】入脾、胃、肺经。

【功用】

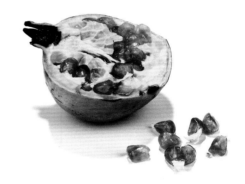

生津止渴。酸石榴兼能涩肠，止血；甜石榴兼能杀虫。适宜于津伤燥渴，久痢滑泻，崩漏带下，虫积等人食用。

【服食方法】

鲜食。

【食宜食忌】

不宜多食。

【储藏】

鲜果放阴凉处保存。

Shi Liu

Pomegranate

【Origin】
　　The fruit of *Punica granatum* L. in the family of Punicaceae.

【Collection / Processing】
　　Collect the ripe fruits during September to October, and use fresh.

【Flavor / Properties】 Sour, sweet, or astringent in flavor, and warm in nature.

【Meridian Tropism】 Spleen, Stomach and Lung.

【Functions and Indications】
　　Promote the production of body fluid to quench thirst. Sour pomegranate fruit can also astringent the intestines and stanch bleeding, and sweet pomegranate fruit can also kill the worms. Recommended for those with body fluid deficiency and thirst, chronic dysentery and chronic diarrhea, uterine bleeding and morbid leucorrhea, or intestinal parasitosis.

【Preparation / Consumption】
　　Use fresh.

【Cautions / Contraindications】
　　Avoid excessive use.

【Storage】
　　Preserve the fresh fruits in shady place.

火龙果
Huo Long Guo

【基原或来源】

为仙人掌科三角柱属植物火龙果*Hylocereus undatus*的果实。

【采收加工或制法】

火龙果在种植12～14个月后开始开花结果，全年可开花12～15次，夏、秋季采摘。选购时以果皮鲜亮紫红，压按果体时软硬适中者为佳。

【性味】 味甘、淡，性凉。

【归经】 入肺、胃、大肠经。

【功用】

清热生津，润肠通便，解毒抗衰。适宜于口干咽燥，口舌生疮，咳嗽痰多，气喘，胃炎，便秘，中暑，重金属中毒，早衰，老年性痴呆，肥胖，高血压，青春痘，痔疮者使用。

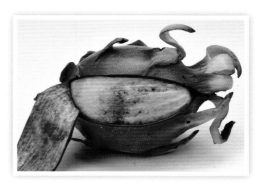

【服食方法】

可生吃、榨汁、凉拌、炒食；制作饮料、酸奶、果冻、果酒、果醋、果脯、冰淇淋等。

【食宜食忌】

脾胃虚寒者、糖尿病患者不宜多食。

【储藏】

宜即买即食；或暂放阴凉、通风处保存。不宜放冰箱贮藏，以防冻伤变质。

Huo Long Guo

Pitaya

【Origin】

It is the fruit of *Hylocereus undatus* of family Cactaceae.

【Collection / Processing】

After being planted for 12~14 months, it flowers and fruits. The plant can flower 12~15 times through the year and people can collect the fruits in summer and autumn. The fruits with bright purplish red peel and proper hardness of the fruit body are of good quality.

【Flavor / Properties】 Sweet and tasteless in flavor, cool in nature.

【Meridian Tropism】 Lung, Stomach and Large Intestine.

【Functions and Indications】

Clear heat and promote fluid production, moisten intestine to relieve constipation, detoxicate and anti-aging. Used for dry mouth and throat, ulcers in mouth, cough with much sputum, short of breath, gastritis, constipation, sun stroke, poisoning with heavy metal, premature aging, senile dementia, obesity, hypertension, acne, hemorrhoids, etc.

【Preparation / Consumption】

Take the fresh fruit, squeeze juice, mix with seasonings, stir-fried, or make drinks, yogurt, jelly, fruit wine, fruit vinegar, candied fruit, ice-cream, etc.

【Cautions / Contraindications】

The one who has deficient-cold of spleen and stomach as well as diabetes should not take it too much.

【Storage】

Take the fresh fruit or it should be preserved in cool and well-ventilated place. It is unadvisable to preserve the fruit in the refrigerator to prevent from frost damage.

榴 莲
Liu Lian

【基原或来源】

为木棉科榴莲属植物榴莲*Durio zibethinus* Murr.的果实。

【采收加工或制法】

为不影响榴莲成熟及果树受到损伤，一般不采摘，而是等其成熟后，在清晨或深夜自落，捡拾即可。购买时以果形完整端正，果皮呈深咖啡色，刺粗大而疏，味道浓烈，摇晃时感觉有物，相邻刺易捏在一起（表明成熟）者为佳。

【性味】性热，味甘。

【归经】入胃、大肠经。

【功用】

温中开胃，散寒止泻。适宜于寒性胃痛，痛经，痢疾，泄泻，高血压，皮肤瘙痒，贫血，乳腺炎，视网膜炎，水肿，骨质疏松者使用。

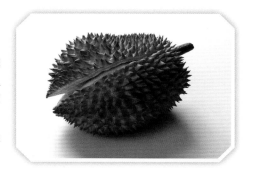

【服食方法】可直接生食，榨汁；煲汤，如榴莲炖鸡；酿酒。

【食宜食忌】

阴虚火旺易口舌生疮者慎食；肥胖者、糖尿病患者慎食。榴莲性热，宜配山竹、西瓜等食用；榴莲果肉黏稠，易结于肠内，故食后宜喝些开水，以助消化；榴莲富含纤维素，在肠胃内会吸水膨胀，可引起便秘，故不宜多食。

【储藏】

放于阴凉、通风处保存。裂开的榴莲可取出果肉，套上保鲜膜放冰箱暂存，食之会有雪糕口感。若闻到有酒精味，则已变质，不可食用。

Liu Lian

Durian

【Origin】 It is the fruit of *Durio zibethinus* Murr. of family Bombacaceae.

【Collection / Processing】

It is better to wait for the ripe fruit drop from the tree and pick it up. The fruit which is complete, with dark brown colored pericarp, bulky and sparse pricks, strongly scented, felt with something inside when shaking, and the adjacent pricks which are easy to knead together (it indicates that the fruit is ripe), is of good quality.

【Flavor / Properties】 Hot in nature and sweet in flavor.

【Meridian Tropism】 Stomach and Large Intestine.

【Functions and Indications】

Warm the middle energizer and promote appetite, disperse cold and check diarrhea. Used for stomachache due to cold, dysmenorrhea, dysentery, diarrhea, hypertension, itching skin, anemia, mastitis, retinitis, edema, osteoporosis, etc.

【Preparation / Consumption】

Take the fresh fruit, squeeze juice, cook soup, e.g. stewed with chicken, or make wine.

【Cautions / Contraindications】

The one who has *yin* deficiency with effulgent fire and oral ulcers, the diabetic and the obese should take it with caution. The fruit is hot in nature and it can be taken with mangosteen and watermelon; its pulp is sticky and is easy to stagnate in the intestine so it is better to drink some water after consumption to promote digestion. However, it should not be taken too much because the fruit is rich in cellulose so it will suck water in the stomach and intestine and become enlarged, thus result in constipation.

【Storage】

Preserved in cool and well-ventilated place. Take out the pulp from the chapped fruit, wrap it with preservative film and put it in the refrigerator for preservation. It will taste like ice-cream when consumption. However, if there is alcoholic odour, it indicates that the fruit is not suitable for consumption.

山 竹
Shan Zhu

【基原或来源】

　　为藤黄科藤黄属植物山竹*Garcinia mangostana*.L.的果实。

【采收加工或制法】

　　秋季采收果实。选购时以蒂绿、果皮较软的新鲜山竹为佳。

【性味】味甘、酸，性凉。

【归经】入肺、脾、大肠经。

【功用】

　　清热泻火，补阴生津，化痰止咳。适宜于口干咽燥，口舌生疮，中暑，肺阴不足，咳嗽痰热，胃火旺盛，胃炎，胃溃疡，便秘，抑郁，失眠，皮肤干燥粗糙，病后体虚者使用。

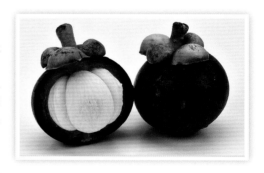

【服食方法】

　　可生吃，榨汁，做沙拉，制作罐头等。山竹果皮味苦涩，剥皮时需防止将果皮汁液染在肉瓣上，以免影响口感。

【食宜食忌】

　　山竹性凉，脾胃虚寒者慎食；也不宜与西瓜、苦瓜等寒凉食物同食。山竹含糖分较高，糖尿病人忌食。

【储藏】

　　可用保鲜膜封好放冰箱暂存或放阴凉、通风处保存。

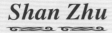

Shan Zhu

Mangosteen

【Origin】

The fruit of *Garcinia mangostana*. L. of *Garcinia* genus in the family of Clusiaceae.

【Collection / Processing】

Collect the fruits in autumn. Tips for purchase: it is advised to choose the fresh one with green pedicle and soft pericarp.

【Flavor / Properties】 Sweet and sour in flavor, cool in nature.

【Meridian Tropism】 Lung, Spleen and Large Intestine.

【Functions and Indications】

Clear heat and reduce fire, invigorate *yin* and regenerate body fluids, relieve cough and reduce sputum. Recommended for those with dry mouth and throat, ulcer in mouth or tongue, heat stroke, insufficiency of lung *yin*, cough with phlegm heat, high stomach-fire, gastritis, gastric ulcer, constipation, depression, insomnia, xerosis cutis and pachycosis, or weakness after disease.

【Preparation / Consumption】

It can be consumed directly, or used to extract juice, make salad or canned goods. The pericarp has a bitter and puckery taste, so caution is needed for peeling to avoid the pericarp juice dye on the pulp, so as not to affect the taste.

【Cautions / Contraindications】

For its cool nature, people with deficiency-cold of spleen and stomach should take it with caution. It cannot be eaten together with some cold food such as watermelon and bitter gourd. It is rich in sugar, so it is contraindicated for people with diabetes.

【Storage】

Stored in shady and ventilated area, or to be sealed up with freshness-keeping plastic film to be temporarily kept in refrigerator.

柚 子
You Zi

【基原或来源】

为芸香科植物柚*Citrus grandis*（L.）Osbeck.的成熟果实。

【采收加工或制法】

秋季果实成熟时采摘。

【性味】味甘、酸，性寒。

【归经】入肝、脾、胃经。

【功用】

消食开胃，化痰醒酒。适宜于食积，食欲不振，妊娠呕吐，咳嗽有痰，醉酒口臭者食用。

【服食方法】

鲜食、绞汁饮服、煮水、熬膏等。

【食宜食忌】

气虚者慎食，服药期间慎食。

【储藏】

放阴凉干燥处保存。

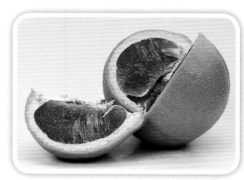

You Zi

Pomelo

【Origin】

The mature fruit of *Citrus grandis* (L.) Osbeck. in the family of Rutaceae.

【Collection / Processing】

Pick when the fruit is mature in autumn.

【Flavor / Properties】 Sweet and sour in flavor, cold in nature.

【Meridian Tropism】 Lung, Spleen and Stomach.

【Functions and Indications】

Promote digestion and appetite, reduce phlegm and dispel the effects of alcohol. Dyspepsia, inappetence, vomiting of pregnancy, cough with phlegm, and drunkenness with bad breath.

【Preparation / Consumption】

It can be taken uncooked, or made into juice, soup or cream.

【Cautions / Contraindications】

Those with insufficient *qi* or in medication period should be cautious to take it.

【Storage】

It should be put in shady, cool and dry place.

樱 桃
Ying Tao

【基原或来源】

为蔷薇科植物樱桃*Prunus pseudocerasus* Lindl.的果实。

【采收加工或制法】

初夏果实成熟时采收。

【性味】 味甘，性温。

【归经】 入脾、肾经。

【功用】

健脾益肾，祛风除湿，通络止痛。适用于风湿痹证，四肢不仁，腰腿疼痛，肾虚遗精，脾虚下利，冻疮痒肿，麻疹难发者使用。

【服食方法】

鲜食，绞汁，或浸酒服。外用：浸酒涂擦或捣敷。

【食宜食忌】

内热、有喘嗽者不可食。

【储藏】

放阴凉或低温处保存。

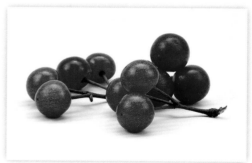

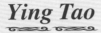

Ying Tao

Cherry

【Origin】
The fruit of *Prunus pseudocerasus* Lindl. in the family of Rosaceae.

【Collection / Processing】
Collect the ripe fruits in the early summer.

【Flavor / Properties】 Sweet in flavor and warm in nature.

【Meridian Tropism】 Spleen and Kidney.

【Functions and Indications】
Invigorate spleen and tonify kidney, dispel wind and eliminate dampness, dredge collaterals to stop pain. Used for arthralgia of wind-damp, insensitivity of the limbs, pain in the lumbus and legs, emission with renal asthenia, diarrhea due to spleen deficiency, itching pain of perniosis, or measles inhabited eruption of.

【Preparation / Consumption】
Use fresh, squeezed into juice, or soaked into wine. External use: inunction after soaked in wine or application after grinded.

【Cautions / Contraindications】
Those with internal heat or panting and cough should not eat it.

【Storage】
Stored in shady and low temperature area.

杨 梅
Yang Mei

【基原或来源】

为杨梅科杨梅属植物杨梅 *Myrica rubra* （Lour．） Sieb．et Zucc．的果实。

【采收加工或制法】

夏季成熟时采摘，鲜用，干用或盐渍备用。

【性味】 味酸、甘，性温，无毒。

【归经】 入脾、胃、肝经。

【功用】

生津止渴，消食和胃，解酒止吐，止血生肌。用于心烦口渴，食欲不振，泄泻痢疾，食积腹痛，酗酒呕吐，头痛衄血。

【服食方法】

生啖、浸酒、腌食。

【食宜食忌】

不宜多食，忌与生葱同食。

【储藏】

腌制晒干或浸酒保存。

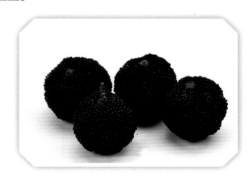

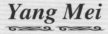

Yang Mei

Waxberry

【Origin】
It's the fruit of *Myrica rubra* (Lour.) Sieb. et Zucc. in the family of Myricaceae.

【Collection / Processing】
Herborized when the fruits are ripe in summer. It can be used when fresh, dry or reserved after salting.

【Flavor / Properties】 Sour and sweet in flavor, warm in nature, and non-toxic.

【Meridian Tropism】 Spleen, Stomach and Liver.

【Functions and Indications】
Promoting the production of body fluid to quench thirst, promoting digestion and regulating stomach, alleviating a hangover and antiemesis, promote tissue regeneration and hemostatic. It is used for upset and thirsty, poor appetite, diarrhea, dyspeptic abdominalgia, vomiting for excessive drinking, headache for non-traumatic hemorrhage.

【Preparation / Consumption】
It can be taken when fresh, or soaked in wine, or preserved by salting.

【Contraindications / Cautions】
It is advisable not to take too much, and it is contraindicated to take together with scallion.

【Storage】
It can be stored by sousing, drying or being soaked in wine.

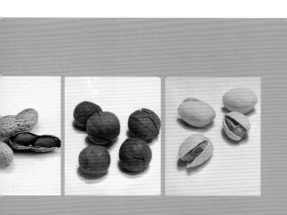

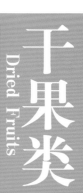

干果类
Dried Fruits

葵花子
Kui Hua Zi

【基原或来源】为菊科向日葵属植物向日葵*Helianthus annuus* L.的种子。

【采收加工或制法】

　　果实成熟后采收，晒干或烘干备用。选材以粒大饱满、壳黑、干燥、无坏粒、无霉烂者为佳。

【性味】味甘，性平。

【归经】入心、肺、大肠经。

【功用】

　　透脓透疹，止痢。适宜于脾胃气虚，食欲不振，虚弱头风，血痢，麻疹透发不畅，痈肿，蛲虫病，便秘者使用。

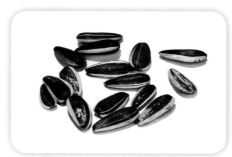

【服食方法】

　　可炒食，制作糕点，榨油等。

【食宜食忌】

　　大便溏薄、肠道功能欠佳者不宜多食。阴虚火旺体质者不宜多食，以免上火，导致口舌生疮。

【储藏】

　　置于干燥容器内密封保存，防潮防蛀。

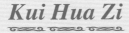

Kui Hua Zi

Sunflower Seed

【Origin】
The seed of *Helianthus annuus* L. of *Helianthus* genus in the family of Compositae.

【Collection / Processing】
Collect the ripe fruits, get them dried or baked. Tips for purchase: full shaped and big sized, shell black, dry, no bad or rotten grains.

【Flavor / Properties】 Sweet in flavor and neutral in nature.

【Meridian Tropism】 Heart, Lung and Large Intestine.

【Functions and Indications】
Outthrust pus and promote eruptions, stop dysentery. Recommended for those with *qi* deficiency of spleen and stomach, poor appetite, weakness and head-wind, bloody flux, obstruction in measles outthrusting, carbuncle, enterobiasis, or constipation.

【Preparation / Consumption】
It can be stir-fried, made into cake, or squeezed into oil.

【Contraindications / Cautions】
Large quantity of consumption is not recommended for those with loose stool, poor function with intestinal tract. To avoid suffering from excessive internal heat that leads to sores in mouth or tongue, those with excessive pyrexia caused by *yin* deficiency should limit the amount of consumption.

【Storage】
Sealed up in dry containers, moisture and moth proofing.

西瓜子仁
Xi Gua Zi Ren

【基原或来源】

　　为葫芦科西瓜属植物西瓜*Citrullus lanatus* (Thunb.) Matsum. et Nakai.的种仁。

【采收加工或制法】

　　夏季食用西瓜时，收集瓜子，洗净晒干，去壳取仁用。

【性味】味甘，性平。

【归经】入肺、胃、大肠经。

【功用】

　　清肺化痰，和中止渴，润肠通便。用于肺热久嗽，咳血吐血，暑热烦渴，肠燥便秘。

【服食方法】

　　生食、炒熟食、煮粥、煮汤饮等。

【食宜食忌】

　　不宜多食。

【储藏】

　　放阴凉干燥处保存。

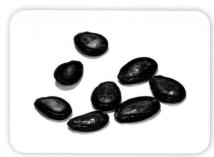

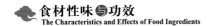

Xi Gua Zi Ren

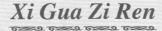

Watermelon Seed Kernel

【Origin】
The seed kernel of *Citrullus Lanatus* (Thunb.) Matsum. et Nakai plant in the family Cucurbitaceae.

【Collection / Processing】
Collect the seeds when eating watermelon in summer, wash and dry in the sun, remove the shell and take out the kernel.

【Flavor / Properties】 Sweet in flavor, neutral in nature.

【Meridian Tropism】 Lung, Stomach and Large Intestine.

【Functions and Indications】
Clear lung and resolve phlegm, harmonize the middle energizer relieve thirsty, moisten and relax bowels. Lung heat, long cough, hemoptysis, hematemesis, polydipsia, dry bowels and constipation.

【Preparation / Consumption】
It can be taken uncooked, fried, or cooked in congee or soup.

【Cautions / Contraindications】
It should not be taken too much.

【Storage】
It should be put in shady, cool and dry place.

胡桃仁
Hu Tao Ren

【基原或来源】

　　为胡桃科胡桃属植物胡桃 *Juglans regia* L．的种仁。

【采收加工或制法】

　　于白露前后果实成熟时采收。

【性味】味甘，性温，无毒。

【归经】入肺、肾、肝经。

【功用】

　　温肺定喘，补肾固精，润肠通便。用于咳嗽气喘，阳痿遗精，腰痛脚弱，尿频石淋，疝气腹痛，肠燥便秘，瘰疬疮疡。

【服食方法】

　　炒食，煮粥，制糕点等。

【食宜食忌】

　　肺有痰热、阴虚火旺者及泄泻、大便溏薄者忌食。

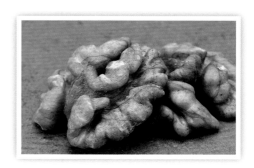

【储藏】

　　本品易返油、虫蛀，立夏前后，须藏于冷室内。

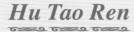

Hu Tao Ren

Walnut

【Origin】
It is the kernel of *Juglans regia* L. in the family of Juglandaceae.

【Collection / Processing】
Herborized around White Dew (15th solar term) when the fruit is ripe.

【Flavor / Properties】 Sweet in flavor, warm in nature and non-toxic.

【Meridian Tropism】 Lung, Kidney and Liver.

【Functions and Indications】
Warm lung to relieve asthma, tonify kidney to control nocturnal emission, moisten intestine to relieve constipation. Commonly used for cough and asthma, impotence and spermatorrhea, lumbago and feeble feet, frequent urination and urolithiasis, abdominal pain due to hernia, constipation due to dryness in the intestine, scrofula, sores and boils, etc.

【Preparation / Consumption】
It can be stir-fried or be used to cook porridge and make desserts, etc.

【Contraindications / Cautions】
It is contraindicated for the one who has phlegm and heat in the lung, excessive fire due to *yin* deficiency, diarrhea and loose stool, etc.

【Storage】
It is liable to bleed with oil and be damaged by moth so that it should be refrigerated around the Beginning of Summer (7th solar term).

落花生
Luo Hua Sheng

【基原或来源】

为豆科落花生属植物落花生*Arachis hypogaea* L.的种子。

【采收加工或制法】

秋末挖取果实，剥去果壳，取种子，晒干。

【性味】 味甘，性平。

【归经】 入脾、肺经。

【功用】

健脾养胃，润肺化痰。适宜于脾虚不运，反胃便秘，乳妇奶少，肺燥咳嗽等病症者食用。

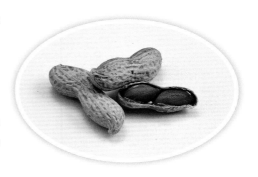

【服食方法】

可生食、凉拌、煮粥、做汤、油炸、炒食等。

【食宜食忌】

体寒湿滞及肠滑便泄者不宜服。

【储藏】

晒干后，置于袋中或罐内密封保存。

Luo Hua Sheng

Peanut

【Origin】
It is the seed of *Arachis hypogaea* L. of *Arachis* plant of family Leguminosae.

【Collection / Processing】
Collect the fruit in late autumn, peel to get the seeds and dry the seeds in the sun.

【Flavor / Properties】 Sweet in flavor and moderate in nature.

【Meridian Tropism】 Spleen and Lung.

【Functions and Indications】
Invigorate spleen and nourish stomach, moisten lung and resolve sputum. Used for disorder of transporting and transforming function due to spleen deficiency, nausea, constipation, lack of breast milk, coughing due to lung dryness, etc.

【Preparation / Consumption】
Take the fresh peanut, mix with seasonings, cook porridge or soup, fried in oil or stir-fried, etc.

【Cautions / Contraindications】
The one who has dampness stagnation due to cold in the body, lubricated intestines and diarrhea should not take it.

【Storage】
Preserved in a bag or container air-tightly after drying in the sun.

山核桃
Shan He Tao

【基原或来源】

为胡桃科山核桃属植物山核桃*Carya cathayensis* Sarg.的核仁。

【采收加工或制法】

秋季果实成熟时采摘，干燥备用，临用时去果皮取仁。或干燥后去皮取仁，密封保存以备用。选材以粒大壳薄、果仁饱满、油脂丰富者为佳。

【性味】味甘，性温。

【归经】入肺、肝、肾经。

【功用】

补益肝肾，纳气平喘。适宜于肝肾亏虚之腰膝酸软无力、腰部隐痛不适，及肺肾不足、肾不纳气之虚咳、久咳、咳之无力者食用。

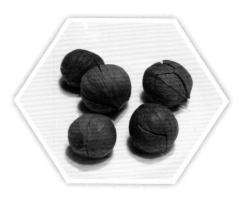

【服食方法】

生食、煮粥、炒食，制作糖果及糕点的佐料，也可榨取山核桃油食用。

【食宜食忌】

盐炒后阴虚火旺体质者不宜多食，以免上火。

【储藏】

置于阴凉干燥处，防潮、防蛀。去皮之果仁应防泛油。

Shan He Tao

Hickory Kernel

【Origin】

The fruit-kernel of *Carya cathayensis* Sarg. in the family of Juglandaceae.

【Collection / Processing】

Collect the ripe fruits in autumn, get them dried, and peel to take out the kernels for use. Or, collect the kernels after the fruits have been dried and peeled, get them sealed up for storage. It is advised to choose the one with big shape, thin shell, full shaped kernel, and abundant in lipid.

【Flavor / Properties】 Sweet in flavor and warm in nature.

【Meridian Tropism】 Lung, Liver and Kidney.

【Functions and Indications】

Tonify the liver and benefit the kidney, promote inspiration to relieve asthma. Recommended for those with the liver-kidney asthenia caused limp aching, weakness of lumbus and knees, lumbar vague pain and discomfort, and the lung-kidney asthenia and the kidney *qi* absorption failure caused vacuity cough, chronic cough, and cough of weakness.

【Preparation / Consumption】

It can be used fresh, boiled into porridge, or stir-fried; it can also be used as accessory food for candy or cake processing, or used to make cathay hickory oil.

【Cautions / Contraindications】

After salty stir-fried, to avoid suffering from excessive internal heat, large quantity of consumption is not advised for those with excessive pyrexia caused by *yin* asthenia.

【Storage】

Stored in shady and ventilated area, moisture and moth proofing. Oil secretion should be prevented for the peeled kernels storage.

杏 仁
Xing Ren

【基原或来源】

为蔷薇科植物杏*Armeniaca vulgaris* Lam.或山杏*Armeniaca sibirica* (L.) Lam.等的种子。

【采收加工或制法】

夏季果实成熟时采摘，除去果肉及核壳，取种仁。

【性味】 味苦，性温，有小毒。

【归经】 入肺、胃、大肠经。

【功用】

祛痰止咳，降气平喘，润肠通便，消食定痛。适宜于外感咳嗽，气喘痰鸣，肠燥便秘，食滞脘痛者食用。

【服食方法】

炒食、煮粥食等。

【食宜食忌】

阴虚燥咳、大便滑泄者慎食或勿食。

【储藏】

置阴凉干燥处，防虫蛀。

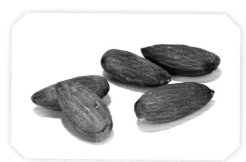

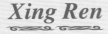

Xing Ren

Apricot Kernel

【Origin】
The seed of *Armeniaca vulgaris* Lam. or *Armeniaca sibirica* (L.) Lam., plant in the family Rosaceae.

【Collection / Processing】
Pick when the fruit is mature in summer, remove the pulp and the nuclear shell, and take the kernel.

【Flavor / Properties】 Bitter in flavor, warm in nature, slightly toxic.

【Meridian Tropism】 Lung, Stomach and Large Intestine.

【Functions and Indications】
Eliminate phlegm and stop cough, direct *qi* downward to relieve asthma, moisten intestines to relax bowels, help digestion and alleviate pain. Cough of external contraction, asthma, gurgling with sputum, dry bowels, constipation, dyspepsia and gastral pain.

【Preparation / Consumption】
It can be fried, or cooked in congee.

【Cautions / Contraindications】
Those with dry cough of insufficient *yin* or loose stool should be cautious to or must not take it.

【Storage】
It should be put in shady, cool and dry place, without damage by worm.

腰 果
Yao Guo

【基原或来源】

为漆树科植物腰果*Anacardium occidentale* L.的果实。

【采收加工或制法】

夏、秋季果实成熟时采收，除去假果，留取核果，晒干。购买时以果体饱满完整、色泽白、气味清香、无斑点、无虫蛀者为佳。

【性味】味甘，性平。

【归经】入肺、脾、肾经。

【功用】

健脾润肺，补肾，止渴。适宜于咳嗽气逆，食欲不佳，口渴者食用。

【服食方法】

可生食、炒食、油炸、做菜肴，或制作蜜饯、糕点、果汁、果酱、果脯、盐渍果仁、果仁糖等。

【食宜食忌】

对腰果过敏者忌食；腰果富含油脂，故胆功能不良者慎食。

【储藏】

宜存放于密闭容器或保鲜袋内密封，置阴凉、干燥处，防潮防蛀。

Yao Guo

Cashew Nut

【Origin】

The fruit of *Anacardium occidentale* L.in the family of Anacardiaceae.

【Collection / Processing】

Harvested in the summer or autumn when the fruit is ripe. Remove the spurious fruits; collect the stone fruits to be dried in the sun. Tips for purchase: it is advised to choose the one with integrated and fleshy body, brightly white color, fragrant smell, no spot and no insect bites.

【Flavor / Properties】 Sweet in flavor, and neutral in nature.

【Meridian Tropism】 Lung, Spleen and Kidney.

【Functions and Indications】

Strengthen the spleen and moisturize the lung, invigorates the kidney, and quench thirst. Recommended for those with cough and *qi* regurgitation, poor appetite, and thirst.

【Preparation / Consumption】

It can be used fresh, stir-fried, oil-fried, or cooked together with other foods. It can also be made into conserves, cakes, fruit juice, fruit jam, preserved fruits, salted nutlet, and praline, etc.

【Cautions / Contraindications】

Those allergic to cashew nut should avoid in eating, and those with gall bladder dysfunction should use with caution because it is rich in fat.

【Storage】

It is advised to stored in hermetic containers or sealed in plastic bags, and placed in cool, dry and moth proofing area.

榧 子
Fei Zi

【基原或来源】

为红豆杉科植物榧树 *Torreya grandis* Fort. ex Lindl.的成熟种子。

【采收加工或制法】

秋季种子成熟时采摘，除去肉质假种皮，洗净，晒干备用。购买时以种仁细小、饱满充实、干燥、无杂质、无虫蛀者为佳。

【性味】味甘、涩，性平。

【归经】入肺、胃、大肠经。

【功用】

消谷，杀虫，通便，润肺止咳。适宜于虫积腹痛，疳积，肺燥咳嗽，肠燥便秘，痔疮肿痛，蛔虫病，钩虫病等使用。

【服食方法】

煎汤，炒熟去壳嚼服，亦可蒸食，代茶饮用，煮羹，或制作成饮料等。

【食宜食忌】

泄泻肠滑者慎食。

【储藏】

放于阴凉干燥处，宜连壳保存，以防虫蛀。

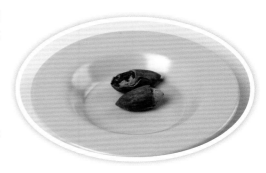

Fei Zi

Chinese Torreya

【Origin】

The ripe seed of *Torreya grandis* Fort. ex Lindl. in the family of Taxaceae.

【Collection / Processing】

The ripe seeds are harvested in the autumn, and ready for use after the pulp aril are removed, cleaned and dried. Tips for purchase: it is recommended for choose the one with small, full and well-stacked, dry seed body, no foreign matters, and no insect bites.

【Flavor / Properties】 Sweet and astringent in flavor, and neutral in nature.

【Meridian Tropism】 Lung, Stomach and Large Intestine.

【Functions and Indications】

Accelerate digestion, kill worms, free the stool, and moisten the lung to arrest cough. It is used to resolve abdominal pain due to helminthic accumulation, malnutrition with accumulation, cough of lung dryness, constipation due to dryness of the intestine, sore pain of piles, ascariasis, and ancylostomiasis, etc.

【Preparation / Consumption】

It can be decocted into soup, stir-fried and eaten after decorticated, steamed, used as tea, or it can also be made into porridge or drinking.

【Cautions / Contraindications】

Use caution for those with diarrhea and lubricated intestines.

【Storage】

Stored in cool and dry area, with integrated shells to prevent moth.

开心果
Kai Xin Guo

【基原或来源】

为漆树科黄连木属落叶小乔木植物阿月浑子 *Pistacia vera* L.的果实。

【采收加工或制法】

7~9月采摘成熟果实。购买时以果仁完整饱满，色泽鲜绿者为佳。

【性味】味辛、甘、微涩，性温。

【归经】入脾、肾、大肠经。

【功用】

温肾助阳，暖脾止痢。适宜于脾肾阳虚，腰际酸冷，阳痿，早泄，冷痢寒泄，身体瘦弱，食欲不振等人使用。

【服食方法】

可生食、炒食、烤、炸、腌制、糖制、榨油；亦可制作成干果、糕点、奶酪、清凉饮料、冰淇淋等。

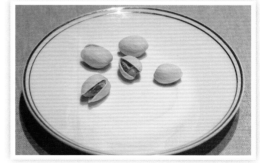

【食宜食忌】

阴虚火旺者不宜多食。

【储藏】

放阴凉、干燥处或冰箱内保存，防霉防蛀。

Kai Xin Guo

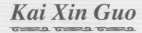

Pistachio Nut

【Origin】
The fruit of the deciduous small tree, *Pistacia vera* L., of *Pistacia* genus in the family of Anacardiaceae.

【Collection / Processing】
Harvest the ripe fruits during July to September. Tips for purchase: it is advised to choose the one with integrated and well-stacked nutlet, and fresh green color.

【Flavor / Properties】 Pungent, sweet, and slightly astringent in flavor, and warm in nature.

【Meridian Tropism】 Spleen, Kidney and Large Intestine.

【Functions and Indications】
Warm kidney and activates *yang*, warm the stomach and stops dysentery.

【Indications】
Recommended for those with spleen-kidney *yang* deficiency, aching and cold in waist, impotence, cold dysentery and cold diarrhea, thinness and weakness, or poor appetite, etc.

【Preparation / Consumption】
It can be eaten fresh, stir-fried, broiled, oil-fried, salted, pickled with sugar, or used to extract oil. It can also be made into dry fruit, cakes, cheese, cooling drink, and ice cream, etc.

【Cautions / Contraindications】
High quantity consumption is not recommended for those with excessive pyrexia due to *yin* deficiency.

【Storage】
Stored in cool, dry area or in refrigerator, mould and moth proofing.

栗 子
Li Zi

【基原或来源】

　　为壳斗科植物板栗 *Castanea mollissima* Bl. 的种仁。

【采收加工或制法】

　　总苞由青色转黄色，微裂时采收，剥出种子。

【性味】味甘、微咸，性温，无毒。

【归经】入肾、脾、胃经。

【功用】

　　健脾养胃，补肾强筋，活血止血，消肿散结。适宜于脾虚泄痢，反胃不食，脚膝酸软，折伤瘀痛，吐衄便血，瘰疬肿毒等。

【服食方法】

　　生食、炒食、煮食、煮粥食。

【食宜食忌】

　　小儿，脾胃虚弱、消化不良者不宜多食。

【储藏】

　　入窖贮藏；或剥出种子，晒干。

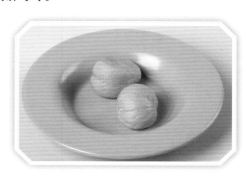

Li Zi

Chestnut

【Origin】
It is the kernel of *Castanea mollissima* Bl. of family Fagaceae.

【Collection / Processing】
Herborized when the involucre is slightly chapped while the color turns to yellow from green. Strip out the seed.

【Flavor / Properties】 Sweet and slightly salty in flavor, warm in nature and non-toxic.

【Meridian Tropism】 Kidney, Spleen and Stomach.

【Functions and Indications】
Invigorate spleen and nourish stomach, tonify kidney and strengthen tendons, activate blood and stop bleeding, diminish swelling and dissipate masses. It is suitable for the one who has diarrhea due to spleen deficiency, regurgitation and anorexia, aching and limp feet and knees stasis pain caused by fracture, hematemesis and hemafecia, or toxin swelling due to scrofula.

【Preparation / Consumption】
Can be taken in the fresh form, or be stir-fried, cooked or be used to make porridge.

【Contraindications / Cautions】
Children and the one who has spleen and stomach deficiency or dyspepsia should not take it too much.

【Storage】
It should be stored in the cellaring or strip out the seed and dry it in the sun.

榛 子
Zhen Zi

【基原或来源】

为桦木科榛属植物榛*Corylus heterophylla* Fisch. ex Bess.的种仁。

【采收加工或制法】

9～10月果实成熟时采摘，去除总苞和果壳等杂质，晾干。购买时以果体较大、饱满而完整，身干，色泽光亮者为佳。

【性味】味甘，性平。

【归经】入肺、脾、胃、肝经。

【功用】

益气开胃，止咳明目。适宜于病后虚弱，食欲不振，心气不足，脾虚泄泻，目视不明，咳嗽，虫积等人食用。

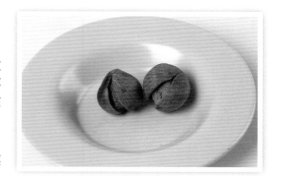

【服食方法】

可生食、煲汤、炒食、蒸食、煮粥、制作糕点、榨油等。

【食宜食忌】

脂肪肝患者、胆功能不良者、易泄泻者慎食。

【储藏】

本品易发油，不宜久存。可用保鲜袋密封，置于阴凉、干燥处暂存，防霉防蛀。

Zhen Zi

Filbert

【Origin】
The seed of *Corylus heterophylla* Fisch. ex Bess. in the family of Betulaceae.

【Collection / Processing】
Harvest the ripe fruit during September to October, remove the impurities as involucre and shell, and then get dried. Tips for purchase: it is advised to choose the one with big, integrated and well-stacked, dry body, and bright color.

【Flavor / Properties】 Sweet in flavor, and neutral in nature.

【Meridian Tropism】 Lung, Spleen, Stomach and Liver.

【Functions and Indications】
Benefit *qi* and promote appetite, relieve cough and improve eyesight. Recommended for those with weakness after illness, poor appetite, deficiency of heart-*qi*, spleen asthenic diarrhea, dim vision, cough, and helminthic accumulation, etc.

【Preparation / Consumption】
It can be used fresh, boiled, stir-fried, steamed, or it can be made into porridge, cakes or squeezed oil.

【Cautions / Contraindications】
Use caution for those with fatty liver, dysfunctional gall bladder, or frequent diarrhea.

【Storage】
It is prone to be oiled, and cannot be store for a long time. It can be sealed up with plastic bag, and placed in cool, dry, mould and moth proofing place for a short time.

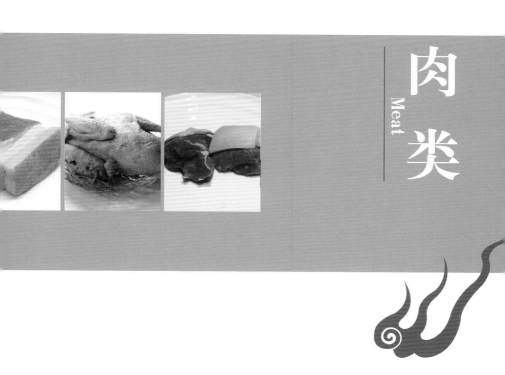

肉 类

Meat

猪 肉
Zhu Rou

【基原或来源】

　　为猪科动物猪 *Sus scrofa domestica* Brisson 的肉。

【采收加工或制法】

　　宰杀后，刮除猪毛，剖腹去内脏，取肉鲜用或冷藏备用。

【性味】味甘、咸，性寒。

【归经】入脾、肾经。

【功用】

　　补肾液，充胃法，滋肝阴，润肌肤。适宜于阴液不足，热病伤津，大便干燥，燥咳无痰，消渴者食用。

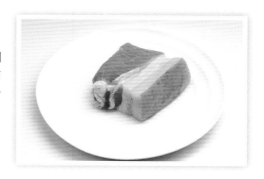

【服食方法】

　　可煮、炖、烧、炒等后食用。

【食宜食忌】

　　湿热、痰滞内蕴者慎服。

【储藏】

　　鲜用、暂冷冻或煮熟之后冷冻保存。

Zhu Rou

Pork

【Origin】

The flesh of *Sus scrofa domestica* Brisson in the family of Suidae.

【Collection / Processing】

Remove the pig hair and internal organs, collect the meat, use fresh or get them cold-stored.

【Flavor / Properties】 Sweet and salty in flavor, cold in nature.

【Meridian Tropism】 Spleen and Kidney.

【Functions and Indications】

Tonify kidney fluids, strengthen stomach, nourish liver *yin*, and moisturize the skin. Recommended for those with insufficiency of *yin*-fluid, consumption of body fluid caused by febrile disease, dry stool, dry cough, or wasting thirst.

【Preparation / Consumption】

Boiled, stewed, roasted, or stir-fried.

【Cautions / Contraindications】

Use caution for those with dampness heat or phlegm stagnation.

【Storage】

Fresh use, or temporarily cold-stored, or cold-stored after it has been cooked.

鸡 肉
Ji Rou

【基原或来源】

为雉科雉属动物家鸡 *Gallus gallus domesticus* Brisson 的肉。

【采收加工或制法】

宰杀后除去羽毛及内脏，取肉鲜用。

【性味】 味甘，性温。

【归经】 归脾、胃经。

【功用】

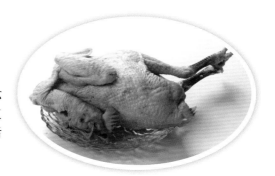

益五脏，补虚损，健脾胃，益精髓。主治虚劳瘦弱，营养不良，病后体虚，食少纳呆，反胃，泻痢，消渴，水肿，及产后乳少等。

【服食方法】

可炖、蒸、煮、烤等后食用，或与其他蔬菜、肉一起炒、炖、炸后食用。

【食宜食忌】

凡患有外感实证邪毒未清及素体痰湿盛者等慎食。

【储藏】

可冷冻或煮熟之后冷冻保存。

Ji Rou

Chicken

【Origin】

It is the meat of *Gallus gallus domesticus* Brisson of family Phasianidae.

【Collection / Processing】

Take the fresh meat after removing the feather and internal organs.

【Flavor / Properties】 Sweet in flavor and warm in nature.

【Meridian Tropism】 Spleen and Stomach.

【Functions and Indications】

It can benefit the five zang organs, tonify the deficient, invigorate spleen and stomach, supplement the essence and marrow. It is used for the consumptive disease, the emaciated, malnutrition, feebleness due to a certain disease, inappetence and anorexia, regurgitation, diarrhea, diabetes, edema, postpartum inadequate breast milk, etc.

【Preparation / Consumption】

It can be stewed, steamed, cooked, and baked, or be stir-fried, stewed and fried with other vegetables or meat.

【Cautions / Contraindications】

The one who has residual evils due to excess syndrome which is caused by external contraction, or the one who always has phlegm and dampness should take chicken carefully.

【Storage】

Cryopreserved directly or cryopreserved after being cooked.

牛 肉
Niu Rou

【基原或来源】

为牛科动物黄牛 *Bos taurus domesticus* Gmelin 或水牛 *Bubalus bubalis* Linnaeus 的肉。

【采收加工或制法】

健康牛宰杀后，剥皮，取肉，水漂洗后，鲜用。

【性味】味甘，性温。

【归经】入脾、胃经。

【功用】

补脾胃，益气血，强筋骨，生津液，止口渴。适宜于脾胃虚弱，气血不足，虚劳羸瘦，消渴，水肿者食用。

【服食方法】

可煮、炖、烧、炒等后食用,或制成牛肉干食用。

【食宜食忌】

牛自死、病死者，禁食其肉；疯牛病肉禁食。

【储藏】

鲜用、暂冷冻或煮熟之后冷冻保存。

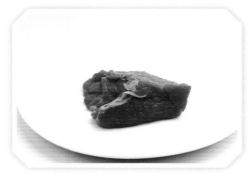

Niu Rou

Beef

【Origin】

The flesh of *Bos taurus domesticus* Gmelin or *Bubalus bubalis* Linnaeus in the family of Bovidae.

【Collection / Processing】

Removes the skin after killing the healthy cattle, collect the meat, clean with water, and use fresh.

【Flavor / Properties】 Sweet in flavor, warm in nature.

【Meridian Tropism】 Spleen and Stomach.

【Function】

Tonify the spleen and stomach, benefit *qi* and blood, strengthen bone and musculature, promote the production of body fluids to quench thirst. Recommended for those with weakness of the spleen and stomach, insufficiency of *qi* and blood, inanition and marked emaciation, wasting thirst, or edema.

【Preparation / Consumption】

Boiled, stewed, roasted, stir-fried, or made into jerky.

【Cautions / Contraindications】

The meat from cow that has died from diseases or other reasons, should not be used for eating. Mad cow meat definitely cannot be used.

【Storage】

Fresh use, or temporarily cold-stored, or cold-stored after it has been cooked.

羊 肉
Yang Rou

【基原或来源】

为牛科动物山羊 *Capra hircus* Linnaeus 或绵羊 *Ovis arise* Linnaeus 的肉。

【采收加工或制法】

取健康羊宰杀后，剥皮，取肉，水漂洗后，鲜用。

【性味】味甘，性温。

【归经】入脾、胃、肾经。

【功用】

补中益气，温中壮阳，滋补强壮。适宜于体质虚弱，阳虚怕冷，手足欠温，胃寒反胃，脘腹冷痛，胃弱不适，肾阳不足，腿脚无力发凉者食用。

【服食方法】

可爆、炒、烤、烧、酱、涮等后食用。

【食宜食忌】

外感时邪或有宿热者禁服；孕妇不宜多食。

【储藏】

鲜用、暂冷冻或煮熟之后冷冻保存。

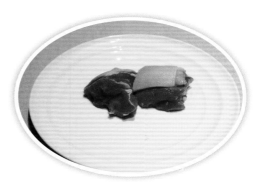

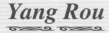

Yang Rou

Mutton

【Origin】
The flesh of *Capra hircus* Linnaeus or *Ovis arise* Linnaeus in the family of Bovidae.

【Collection / Processing】
Remove the skin after killing the healthy sheep, collect the meat, clean them with water, and use fresh.

【Flavor / Properties】 Sweet in flavor, and warm in nature.

【Meridian Tropism】 Spleen, Stomach and Kidney.

【Functions and Indications】
Strengthen the middle energizer and benefit *qi*, warm the middle energizer to strengthen *yang*, tonify and strengthens the body. Recommended for those with weak constitution, fear of cold due to *yang* deficiency, limbs cold, regurgitation due to stomach cold, abdominal crymodynia, dyspepsia, insufficiency of kidney *yang*, or weakness and cold of legs.

【Preparation / Consumption】
It can be quick-fried, stir-fried, grilled, roasted, soused, instantly boiled.

【Cautions / Contraindications】
Contraindicated for those with intrinsic heat and who have diseases caused by exogenous seasonal pathogenic factor. Pregnant women should limit the amount of intake.

【Storage】
Fresh use, or temporarily cold-stored, or cold-stored after it has been cooked.

鸭 肉
Ya Rou

【基原或来源】

为鸭科动物家鸭 *Anas domestica* Linnaeus 的肉。

【采收加工或制法】

四季均可宰杀，除去羽毛及内脏，取肉鲜用。

【性味】味甘、微咸，性凉。

【归经】入肺、脾、肾经。

【功用】

补虚，滋阴，利水。适宜于阴虚体弱或阴虚火旺，虚劳骨蒸，咳嗽，水肿者食用。

【食宜食忌】

患外感，脾胃虚寒，胃腹冷痛，腹泻，或女子经期、肠风下血者禁食或慎食。

【储藏】

鲜食或暂冷冻或煮熟之后冷冻保存。

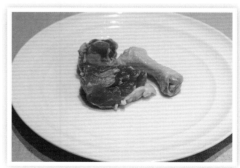

Ya Rou

Duck Meat

【Origin】
The meat of *Anas domestica* Linnaeus in the family of Anatidae.

【Collection / Processing】
Kill in four seasons, remove the feather and the internal organs, and take the meat for fresh use.

【Flavor / Properties】 Sweet and saltish in flavor, cool in nature.

【Meridian Tropism】 Lung, Spleen and Kidney.

【Functions and Indications】
Reinforce insufficiency, nourish *yin*, and induce diuresis. Weakness or effulgent fire with *yin* deficiency, consumptive disease and steaming bone, cough and edema.

【Cautions / Contraindications】
Those with external infection, insufficient-cold spleen and stomach, stomach and abdomen crymodynia, diarrhea or colitis with blood and woman in menstrual period must not or should be cautious to take it.

【Storage】
It should be taken fresh, frozen temporarily, or frozen for storage after being cooked.

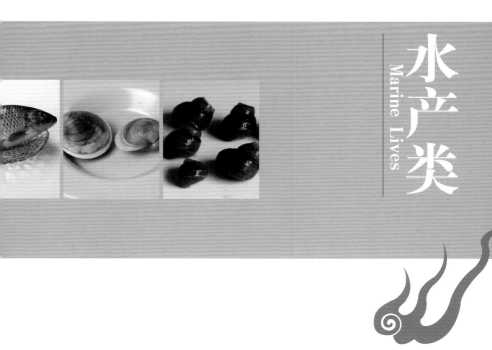

水产类
Marine Lives

鲫 鱼
Ji Yu

【基原或来源】

为鲤科鲫鱼属动物鲫鱼 *Carassius auratus* Linnaeus。

【采收加工或制法】

四季捕捞，除去鳞、鳃及内脏，鲜用。

【性味】味甘，性平，无毒。

【归经】入脾、胃、大肠经。

【功用】

健脾和胃，行水消肿，和血止痢，疗疮平疳。用于反胃吐食，脾胃虚弱，产后乳汁不行，水肿，痈肿，瘰疬，痢疾，便血，牙疳。

【服食方法】

煨汤，红烧，煮食。

【食宜食忌】

鲫鱼平补，诸无所忌。

【储藏】鲜用。

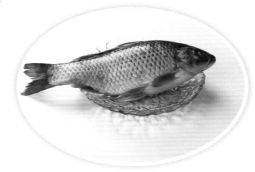

Ji Yu

Crucian

【Origin】
It is a species of Crucian genus in the family of Cyprinidae.

【Collection / Processing】
Caught or harvest all year round, and cooked when fresh, after scales, gill and internal organs are removed.

【Flavor / Properties】 Sweet in flavor, moderate in nature, and nontoxic.

【Meridian Tropism】 Spleen, Stomach and Large Intestine.

【Functions and Indications】
Strengthen the spleen and stomach, promote the normal water flow in the body, subsides swelling, stop bleeding and diarrhea, and cure sore ad malnutrition. Used to resolve regurgitation and throwing up, weakness of the spleen and stomach, lack of lactation after delivery, edema, swelling, scrofula, dysentery, bloody stool, and ulcerative gingivitis.

【Preparation / Consumption】
It can be braised into soup, braised in soy sauce, or boiled.

【Cautions / Contraindications】
Mild tonification, with no contraindications.

【Storage】
Fresh consumption is advised.

带 鱼
Dai Yu

【基原或来源】

为带鱼科带鱼属动物带鱼 *Trichiurus haumela*。

【采收加工或制法】

四季皆可捕捞，洗净，鲜用。

【性味】味甘，性温。

【归经】入肝、胃经。

【功用】

补虚和中，养肝止血，解毒。适宜于久病体虚，食少，产后乳汁不足，胁痛，外伤出血，疮疖等人食用。

【服食方法】

可蒸、烧、煮食。亦可制作咸干制品。

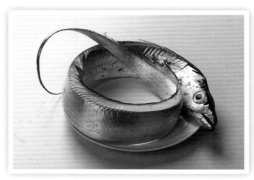

【食宜食忌】

不宜多食。

【储藏】

多鲜食；腌干制品置阴凉通风处。

Dai Yu

Hairtail

【Origin】
Animal of Hairtail genus in the family of Trichiurus.

【Collection / Processing】
Can be caught all year round, and should be cooked fresh after it has been cleaned.

【Flavor / Properties】 Sweet in flavor and warm in nature.

【Meridian Tropism】 Liver and Stomach.

【Functions and Indications】
Tonify deficiency and regulate the middle energizer, nourish liver and stop bleeding, and neutralize poison. Recommended for those with weakness due to chronic disease, poor appetite, lack of lactation after delivery, hypochondrium pain, bleeding wound, sore and furuncle.

【Preparation / Consumption】
Steamed, fried, boiled, or made into salty dried products.

【Cautions / Contraindications】
Frequent use and consumption of high quantities is not recommended.

【Storage】
Consumed fresh, and the salty dried products should be kept in shady and ventilating places.

鲈 鱼
Lu Yu

【基原或来源】

为真鲈科真鲈属动物鲈鱼 *Lateolabrax japonicus* Cuvier et Valenciennes。

【采收加工或制法】

四季均可捕捞。捕获后，除去鳞片及内脏，洗净，鲜用或晒干。

【性味】味甘，性平。

【归经】入肝、脾、肾经。

【功用】

滋肝肾，益脾胃，强筋骨，止咳，安胎。用治脾虚胃痛，消化不良，泄泻，疳积，水肿，痹痛，筋骨萎弱，胎动不安，百日咳等。

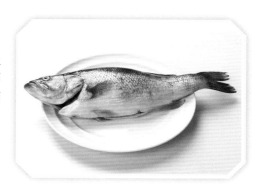

【服食方法】

可蒸、煮、煨、炖等食之。

【食宜食忌】

患皮肤疾患者慎食。

【储藏】

多鲜食；或腌为干制品，贮于阴凉干燥处。

Lu Yu

Perch

【Origin】
  Lateolabrax japonicus Cuvier et Valenciennes of the *Lateolabrax* genus in the family of Percichthyidae.

【Collection / Processing】
  The fish can be caught in all seasons. It can be cooked fresh or dried, after it has been cleaned and the scales and internal organs have been removed.

【Flavor / Properties】 Sweet in flavor and moderate in nature.

【Meridian Tropism】 Liver, Spleen and Kidney.

【Functions and Indications】
  Enrich the liver and kidney, boost the spleen and stomach, strengthen bones and muscles, stop coughing, and prevent miscarriage. Used to resolve spleen asthenia and stomachache, dyspepsia, diarrhea, malnutritional stagnation, edema, impediment, weakness of bones and muscles, fetal irritability, and whooping cough.

【Preparation / Consumption】
  Steamed, boiled, stewed, or braised.

【Cautions / Contraindications】
  Use caution for those with skin diseases.

【Storage】
  Usually eaten fresh, or pickled into dried food, and placed in shady and dry places.

鳝 鱼
Shan Yu

【基原或来源】

为合鳃科鳝属动物黄鳝 *Monopterus albus* Zuiew。

【采收加工或制法】

可采用笼捕、网捕、钓捕等方法捕捉。多鲜食或加工成罐头、鱼干等。

【性味】味甘，性温，无毒。

【归经】入肝、脾、肾三经。

【功用】

补气养血，滋养肝肾，壮筋骨，祛风除湿。用治气血劳伤，腰膝酸软，阳痿，产后恶露不尽，风寒湿痹，下痢脓血，臁疮，痔瘘。

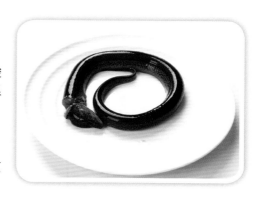

【服食方法】

可炒、爆、炸、烧，或与鸡、鸭、猪等肉类清炖，还可做为火锅原料之一。

【食宜食忌】

患外感、瘙痒性皮肤病及有哮喘等痼疾者慎食。

【储藏】

用鲜品，不宜久贮。

Shan Yu

Eel

【Origin】
It is the animal of family Symbranchidae.

【Collection / Processing】
The eel can be caught by cage, net or fishing, etc. And fresh consumption is advised. However, it also can be processed as cans or dried fish, etc.

【Flavor / Properties】 Sweet in flavor, warm in nature and non-toxic.

【Meridian Tropism】 Liver, Spleen and Kidney.

【Functions and Indications】
Tonify *qi* and nourish blood, nourish liver and kidney, strengthen the tendons and bones, expel wind and resolve dampness. Used for *qi* an blood deficiency, overexertion, lumbar debility, impotence, endless lochia, pain due to wind, cold and dampness, diarrhea with purulent blood, ecthyma and hemorrhoid complicated with anal fistula.

【Preparation / Consumption】
It can be stir-fried, quick-fried, deep-fried, roasted, or boiled in clear soup with chicken, duck or pork, or cooked in the hotpot, etc.

【Cautions / Contraindications】
The one who has exterior syndrome, itchy skin disease, asthma and any chronic illness should take the eel with caution.

【Storage】
It is not suitable for long-time preservation and fresh consumption is advised.

虾
Xia

〰️

【基原或来源】

为长臂虾科沼虾属动物日本沼虾 *Macrobrachium nipponense* de Haan 等。

【采收加工或制法】

5月和11月捕捉，捕获后，洗净鲜用。

【性味】味甘，性温。

【归经】入肝、胃、肾经。

【功用】

补肾壮阳，祛痰托毒，通乳。用治肾虚阳痿，乳汁稀少，麻疹透发不畅，阴疽，恶核，疮痈，丹毒。

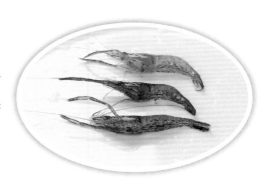

【服食方法】

可炒、煮、烧食等。

【食宜食忌】

对虾过敏者、湿热泻痢、疥癫疮疡者慎食。

【储藏】

鲜活者可放于20℃～30℃的偏碱性的水中暂养；也可用开水或油余一下后，再放入冰箱冷藏，可保持鲜味持久。

Xia

Shrimp

【Origin】

It is the *Macrobrachium nipponense* de Haan of family Palaemonidae.

【Collection / Processing】

It can be caught in May and November. Clean it for fresh consumption.

【Flavor / Properties】 Sweet in flavor and moderate in nature.

【Meridian Tropism】 Liver, Stomach and Kidney.

【Functions and Indications】

Tonify kidney and strengthen *yang*, expel phlegm and promote pus discharge, promote lactation. Used for impotence due to kidney deficiency, scanty breast milk, failure of measles promotion, *yin* furuncles, obstinate nodule, ulcers and carbuncles, erysipelas.

【Preparation / Consumption】

It can stir-fried, boiled or roasted.

【Cautions / Contraindications】

The one who is allergic to shrimp or has diarrhea and dysentery due to dampness and heat, or scabies, favus, ulcers and sores should take it with caution.

【Storage】

Live shrimp can be raised in weak alkaline water which is about 20°C~30°C, or refrigerate the shrimp after being quick-boiled in the boiling water or oil.

蟹
Xie

【基原或来源】

　　为梭子蟹科梭子蟹属三疣梭子蟹 *Portunus trituberculatus*、远海梭子蟹 *Portunus pelagicus*，梭子蟹科蟳属斑纹蟳 *Charybdis feriatus*，梭子蟹科青蟹属锯缘青蟹 *Scylla serrata*，馒头蟹科馒头蟹属卷折馒头蟹 *Calappa lophos*、馒头蟹科虎头蟹属中华虎头蟹 *Orithyia sinica*，蛙蟹科蛙形蟹属蛙形蟹 *Ranina ranina* 等的肉。

【采收加工或制法】

　　每年的九或十月份采捕。

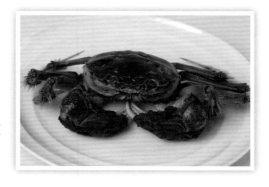

【性味】 味咸，性寒。

【归经】 入肝、胃、肾经。

【功用】

　　清热利湿，退黄，解毒散瘀，消肿。可用于黄疸，产后血瘀腹痛，痈肿疔毒，跌打损伤，漆疮，烫伤等。

【服食方法】

　　可炒，烧，焗，蒸，煮，制羹，煎汤，酒醉，酱渍等。

【食宜食忌】

　　不宜单食；食用时宜去掉螃蟹的鳃、沙包、内脏；死蟹勿食；平素脾胃虚寒，大便溏薄者慎食；不宜与茶水、柿子、兔肉等寒凉食物同食；体质过敏的人、月经期女子及孕妇不宜食。

【储藏】

　　用鲜品。

Xie

Crab

【Origin】

It is the meat of *Portunus trituberculatus* or *Portunus pelagicus* of *Portunus* animal of family Portumidae, or the meat of *Charybdis feriatus* of *Charybdis* of family Portumidae, *Scylla serrata* of *Scylla* animal of family Portumidae, *Calappa lophos* of *Calappa* genus or *Orithyia sinica* of *Orithyia* genus in the family of Calappidae, *Ranina ranina* of *Ranina* genus in the family of Raninidae, etc.

【Collection / Processing】

Catch the crab in September or October every year.

【Flavor / Properties】 Salt in flavor and cold in nature.

【Meridian Tropism】 Liver, Stomach and Kidney.

【Functions and Indications】

Clear heat and drain damp, relieve jaundice, detoxicate and eliminate blood stasis, subside the swelling. Used for jaundice, postpartum abdominal pain due to blood stasis, carbuncles, swelling and furuncles, injuries from falls, fractures and contusions, dermatitis rhus and scalding, etc.

【Preparation / Consumption】

It can be stir-fried, braised, baked, steamed, cooked or used to make thick soup or soup, drunk or sauced, etc.

【Cautions / Contraindications】

It is not suitable to take the crab alone. For consumption, remove its gills, sand sack and internal organs. Don't take the dead crab and the one who has deficient cold of spleen and stomach or loose stool should take it with caution. Besides, it is not suitable to take the crab with cold food such as tea, persimmon and rabbit, etc. And the one who has allergic constitution, woman in menstrual period and the pregnant woman should not eat the crab.

【Storage】

Fresh consumption is advised.

淡 菜
Dan Cai

【基原或来源】

为贻贝科贻贝属动物紫贻贝 *Mytilus edulis* Linnaeus、翡翠贻贝 *Mytilus viridis* Linnaeus及其他贻贝类的肉。

【采收加工或制法】

全年捕采，采获后，剥取其肉，洗净鲜用或加工晒干。

【性味】 味甘、咸，性温。

【归经】 入肝、肾经。

【功用】

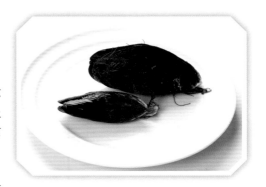

补益肝肾，益精血，消瘿瘤，止崩。适宜于虚劳羸瘦，气血不足，眩晕，盗汗，阳痿，腰痛，吐血，女子崩漏，带下，瘿瘤者等食用。

【服食方法】

可煲汤、蒸、炒、煮食，或与其他菜混炒。

【食宜食忌】

食海鲜类过敏者慎食。

【储藏】

一般多煮熟后加工成干品保存；也可放入水池或盆中暂养（池内须充气，保持水流畅通）。

Dan Cai

Mussel

【Origin】
Flesh of *Mytilus edulis* Linnaeus, *Mytilus viridis* Linnaeus or other *Mytilus* genus animals in the family of Mussels.

【Collection / Processing】
Caught or harvest all year round. Collect the meat after unshelled, and should be eaten or cooked when fresh or dried.

【Flavor / Properties】 Sweet and salty in flavor, and moderate in nature.

【Meridian Tropism】 Liver and Kidney.

【Functions and Indications】
Reinforce liver and benefits kidney, tonify blood and essence, disperse gall-tumor, and stop metrorrhagia. Recommended for those with weakness due to consumption diseases, insufficiency of vital energy and blood, dizziness, night sweat, impotence, low back pain, hematemesis, female uterine bleeding, morbid leucorrhea, and gall-tumor.

【Preparation / Consumption】
Can be made into soup, steamed, fried, boiled, or cooked with other foods.

【Cautions / Contraindications】
Use caution for those allergic to sea foods.

【Storage】
Usually preserved by dried products after cooked, or can temporarily keep alive in water (should flow and be aired).

蛤 蜊
Ge Li

【基原或来源】

为蛤蜊科蛤蜊属动物四角蛤蜊 *Mactra quadrangularis* Deshayes 等的肉。

【采收加工或制法】

全年可采捕。

【性味】味咸，性寒，无毒。

【归经】入胃、肝、膀胱经。

【功用】

滋阴，化痰，软坚，利水，解酒，止消渴。用治消渴，水肿，痰积，癖块，瘿瘤，痔疮，饮酒过度等。

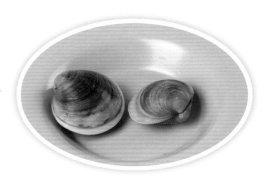

【服食方法】

可炒食、煮食或煨汤。

【食宜食忌】

脾胃虚寒者忌食；女子经期慎食。

【储藏】

蛤蜊宜用淡盐水暂养或放于冰箱冷藏；干品宜贮于阴凉通风干燥处。

Ge Li

Clam

【Origin】
The flesh of *Mactra quadrangularis* Deshayes in the family of Mactridae.

【Collection / Processing】
Caught or harvest all year round.

【Flavor / Properties】 Salty in flavor, cold in nature, and nontoxic.

【Meridian Tropism】 Stomach, Liver and Bladder.

【Functions and Indications】
Nourish *yin*, eliminate sputum, soften hard mass, alleviate water retention, alleviate a hangover, and stop wasting thirst. Used to resolve wasting thirst, edema, phlegm accumulation, aggregation lumps, gall, piles, and intemperance.

【Preparation / Consumption】
Fried, boiled or decocted.

【Cautions / Contraindications】
Contraindicated for those with deficiency cold of spleen and stomach, and use caution during menstruation.

【Storage】
It is advised to keep alive in light salt water or keep fresh in refrigerator. The dried should be kept in shady and air seasoning places.

干 贝
Gan Bei

【基原或来源】

　　为扇贝科栉孔扇贝属动物栉孔扇贝 *Chlamys farreri*、华贵栉孔扇贝 *Chlamys nobilis* 和花鹊栉孔扇贝 *Chlamys pica* 的闭壳肌的干制品。

【采收加工或制法】

　　捕获扇贝后，剥壳，去肉取闭壳肌，洗净煮沸数分钟后取出，洗去黏液，晒干。食用选材以干燥、颗粒完整、大小均匀、呈淡黄色而略有光泽者为佳。

【性味】味甘、咸，性平。

【归经】入脾、胃、肾经。

【功用】

　　滋阴养血，和胃补肾。适宜于久病体虚，消渴，肾虚腰痛，尿频，宿食积滞，食欲不振，气血不足，消化不良者使用。

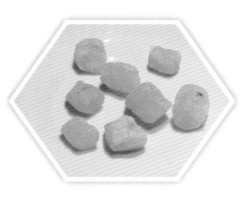

【服食方法】

　　可煲汤、煮粥、作脯、扣炖、蒸食等。

【食宜食忌】

　　脾胃虚弱，气血不足，久病体弱，五脏虚损等病症宜食。尤适宜于咽干口渴，糖尿病，干燥综合征等病症。一次食用量不宜过大。痛风患者不宜食。

【储藏】

　　存放在阴凉处或冰箱冷藏。

Gan Bei

Dried Scallop Adductor

【Origin】

The dried adductor of *Chlamys farreri*, *Chlamys nobilis* and *Chlamys pica* of *Chlamys* genus in the family of Pectenidae.

【Collection / Processing】

Collect the scallops, remove the shells to take out the adductors, make it clean and get it boiled in hot water for a few minutes, get rid of the mucus, and get it dried. Tips for purchase: the high quality dried scallop adductors is dry, full shaped, even sized, and with yellowish luster.

【Flavor / Properties】 Sweet and salty in flavor, neutral in nature.

【Meridian Tropism】 Spleen, Stomach and Kidney.

【Functions and Indications】

Nourish *yin* and blood, regulate the stomach and tonify the kidney. Recommended for those with weakness due to chronic disease, wasting thirst, lumbago due to deficiency of the kidney, frequent micturition, food accumulation, poor appetite, insufficiency of *qi* and blood, or dyspepsia.

【Preparation / Consumption】

Boiled into soup, made into porridge, used as dried meat, stewed, or steamed.

【Cautions / Contraindications】

Recommended for those with weakness of spleen and stomach, insufficiency of *qi* and blood, weakness due to chronic disease, or five organs consumptive disease, particularly for those with dry pharynx and thirst, diabetes, or Sjogren syndrome. It is not advised to consume the dried scallop adductors with a large quantity at one sitting. Those with gout should avoid in eating it.

【Storage】

Stored in shady area or refrigerator.

海 蜇
Hai Zhe

【基原或来源】

为根口水母科海蜇属动物海蜇 *Rhopilema esculenta* Kishinouye 或黄斑海蜇 *Rhopilema hispidum* Vanhoeffen 的口腕部。

【采收加工或制法】

每年8～10月间，海蜇常成群浮游于海上，可用网捕捞。捕获后，将口腕部加工成海蜇头食用。

【性味】味咸，性平，无毒。

【归经】入肺、肝、肾经。

【功用】

平肝清热，化痰消积，润肠通便。用治肺热、痰热咳嗽，哮喘，疳积痞胀，大便燥结，高血压病。

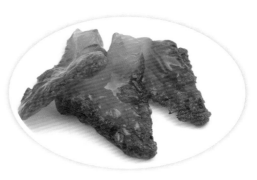

【服食方法】

煮、凉拌或炒食。

【食宜食忌】

脾胃虚寒者慎食。

【储藏】

宜泡于盐水中，放置于阴凉处。

Hai Zhe

Jellyfish

【Origin】

The oral arms of *Rhopilema esculenta* Kishinouye and *Rhopilema hispidum* Vanhoeffen of *Rhopilema* genus in the family of Rhizostomatidae.

【Collection / Processing】

Schools of jellyfish usually float on the sea during August to October, and can be caught by fishing net. After collection, take the oral arms to be manufactured into jellyfish head.

【Flavor / Properties】 Salty in flavor, moderate in nature, and nontoxic.

【Meridian Tropism】 Lung, Liver and Kidney.

【Functions and Indications】

Pacify liver and clear heat, dissipate phlegm to remove food retention, and loosen bowel to relieve constipation. Used to resolve lung-heat, phlegm-heat and cough, asthma, abdominal distention due to malnutritional stagnation, dry feces, and hypertensive disease.

【Preparation / Consumption】

Boiled, fried, or consumption cold, dressed with sauce.

【Cautions / Contraindications】

Use caution for those with deficiency-cold of spleen and stomach.

【Storage】

It is advised to be soaked in salt water and shadily placed.

螺 蛳
Luo Si

【基原或来源】

　　为田螺科环棱螺属动物方形环棱螺 *Bellamya quadrata* 及其同属动物的全体。

【采收加工或制法】

　　四季捕捉。洗净用。

【性味】味甘，性寒。

【归经】入肝、胃、膀胱经。

【功用】

　　清热解毒，利水消肿，止渴，明目。适用于黄疸，水肿，痢疾，疮肿，热淋，消渴，目赤翳障，痔疮者等食用。

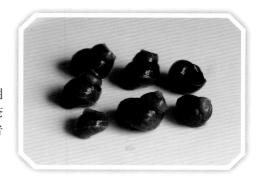

【服食方法】

　　可煮、炒等食之。

【食宜食忌】

　　风寒感冒未愈、脾虚便溏、胃寒者及女子经期、妇人产后忌食。

【储藏】

　　放于清水暂养，一天换一次水。

Luo Si

Spiral Shell

【Origin】

The body of animals as *Bellamya quadrata* of the *Bellamya* genus in the family of Viviparidae.

【Collection / Processing】

Caught in all seasons, and should be cooked after cleaned.

【Flavor / Properties】 Sweet in flavor and cold in nature.

【Meridian Tropism】 Liver, Stomach and Bladder.

【Functions and Indications】

Clear heat and relieve toxicity, and induce diuresis to alleviate edema, slake thirst, and improve eyesight. Recommended for those with jaundice, edema, dysentery, swollen sore, heat strangury, wasting-thirst, conjunctival congestion of eye screen, and haemorrhoids.

【Preparation / Consumption】

Boiled or stir-fried.

【Cautions / Contraindications】

Contraindicated for those with wind-cold type of common cold, loose stool due to spleen asthenia, stomach cold, and women in menstrual period or after childbirth.

【Storage】

Keep alive in clean water, and change the water once in each day.

昆 布
Kun Bu

【基原或来源】

为海带科海带属植物海带 *Laminaria japonica* Aresch. 或翅藻科植物昆布 *Ecklonia kurome* Okam. 的叶状体。

【采收加工或制法】

夏、秋季采捞，洗去杂质，鲜用或晒干用。选购时以整洁干净、无泥沙杂质、无霉变、叶宽厚、色暗绿或黄褐、手感不黏者为佳。

【性味】 味咸、微甘，性寒、滑。

【归经】 入肝、胃、肾、膀胱经。

【功用】

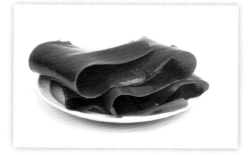

破结软坚，利水消肿。适宜于瘰疬、瘿瘤、颈部淋巴结肿大、甲状腺肿大，面肿，水肿，痰饮，睾丸肿大，奔豚，痈肿瘘疮，食疳，疝瘕，脚气，高血压，肥胖症，皮肤粗糙瘙痒，脑水肿，乳腺增生者使用。

【服食方法】

可凉拌，炒食，炖排骨、炖鸡，做汤，煮粥，腌渍等。

【食宜食忌】

孕妇、产后妇女、脾胃虚寒易泄泻者不宜多食。

【储藏】

宜尽早食用或放冰箱暂存；亦可制成干品保存。

Kun Bu

Kelp

【Origin】

The thallus of *Laminaria japonica* Aresch. of *Laminaria* genus in the family of Laminariaceae or *Ecklonia kurome* Okam. in the family of Alariaceae.

【Collection / Processing】

Collect in summer or autumn, clean to get rid of the foreign matters, and use fresh or get it dried. Tips for purchase: it is advised to choose the one with clean and neat appearance, no foreign matters and mould, broad and thick leaves, dark green or brown color, and non-stick texture.

【Flavor / Properties】 Salty and slightly sweet in flavor, cold and lubricated in nature.

【Meridian Tropism】 Liver, Stomach, Kidney and Bladder.

【Functions and Indications】

Loosen knots and soften hardness, induce diuresis to alleviate edema. Recommended for those with scrofula, gall, cervical lymphadenopathy, goiter, facial swelling, edema, phlegm fluid retention, testicular swelling, up-rushing of *qi*, carbuncle and fistula sores, malnutrition due to improper feeding, mounting-conglomeration, beriberi, hypertension, obesity, rough and itching skin, brain edema, hyperplasia of mammary glands.

【Preparation / Consumption】

It can be used for salad, stir-fried, stewed with sparerib or chicken, made into soup or porridge, or pickled.

【Cautions / Contraindications】

Large quantity of consumption is not recommended for women who are pregnant or after childbirth, or those with deficiency-cold of spleen and stomach and prone to have diarrhea.

【Storage】

Fresh consumption is advised, and it can be temporarily kept in refrigerator. It can also be dried for storage.

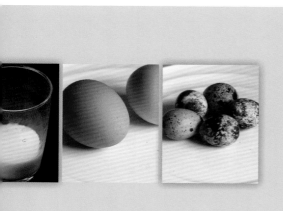

乳蛋类
Milk and Eggs

牛 乳
Niu Ru

【基原或来源】

为母牛乳腺中分泌的乳汁。

【采收加工或制法】

取奶牛乳汁，消毒后鲜用或冷藏。

【性味】味甘，性微寒。

【归经】入心、肺、胃经。

【功用】

补益肺胃，养血润燥。适宜于体质虚弱，气血不足，营养不良，便秘者食用。

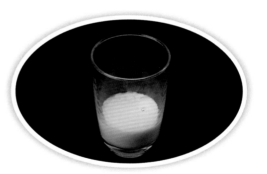

【服食方法】

煮后饮，或煮粥、入膳、做制糕点的辅料等。

【食宜食忌】

脾胃虚寒作泻、中有冷痰积饮者慎服。

【储藏】

宜冰箱中冷藏或制成各种奶制品。

Niu Ru

Cow's Milk

【Origin】
It is the milk secreted from the cow's breast.

【Collection / Processing】
Sterilize the milk for fresh consumption or refrigeration.

【Flavor / Properties】 Sweet in flavor and slightly cold in nature.

【Meridian Tropism】 Heart, Lung and Stomach.

【Functions and Indications】
Tonify lung and stomach, nourish blood and moisten dryness. Used for asthenia, deficient *qi* and blood, malnutrition, constipation, etc.

【Preparation / Consumption】
Take the milk after being boiled, cook porridge or make cakes, etc.

【Cautions / Contraindications】
The one who has deficiency-cold of spleen and stomach or accumulation of cold phlegm in the middle energizer should take it with caution.

【Storage】
Preserved in a refrigerator or make into various kinds of dairy products.

鸡 蛋
Ji Dan

【基原或来源】

为雉科动物家鸡 *Gallus gallus domesticus* Brisson 的卵。

【采收加工或制法】

取鸡蛋鲜用或加工成咸蛋等。

【性味】性平，味甘。

【归经】入心、肺、脾经。

【功用】

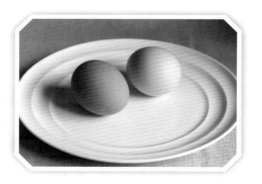

滋阴润燥，健脑安神，养血安胎。适宜于体质素虚，营养不良，气血两虚，妊娠胎动不安，及产后病后调养者食用。

【服食方法】

可煮、炖、烧、炒、腌等后食用。

【食宜食忌】

外感发热、痰饮较盛、食积内停者慎食。

【储藏】

鲜用，腌后或置冰箱中冷藏。

Ji Dan

Chicken Egg

【Origin】

The egg of *Gallus gallus domesticus* Brisson in the family of Phasianidae.

【Collection / Processing】

Collect the eggs, use fresh or be processed into salt eggs.

【Flavor / Properties】 Neutral in nature and sweet in flavor.

【Meridian Tropism】 Heart, Lung and Spleen.

【Functions and Indications】

Nourish *yin* and moisturize dryness-syndrome, invigorate the brain and calms the nerves, nourish blood and prevent abortion. Used for chronic constitution weakness, malnutrition, *qi*-blood deficiency, fetal irritability during pregnancy, or health recovery after child birth or disease.

【Preparation / Consumption】

Boiled, braised, roasted, stir-fried, or pickled.

【Cautions / Contraindications】

Use caution for those with fever caused by exogenous pathogens, severe phlegm-rheum, or abiding food.

【Storage】

Fresh consumption is advised. For storage, it can be pickled, or cold-stored in refrigerator.

鸭 蛋
Ya Dan

【基原或来源】

为鸭科动物家鸭 *Anas domstica* Linnaeus 的卵。

【采收加工或制法】

取鸭蛋鲜用，或加工成咸蛋、皮蛋。

【性味】 味甘，性凉。

【归经】 入肺、大肠经。

【功用】

滋阴、清肺、止泻。适宜于肺热病人咳嗽，咽喉疼痛，热泻下痢者食用。

【服食方法】

可煮、炖、炒、烩、煎或加工成咸蛋、皮蛋等后食用。

【食宜食忌】

不宜多食；脾阳不足，寒湿泻痢，以及食后气滞痞闷者禁食。

【储藏】

鲜用，或宜冰箱中冷藏，或加工成咸蛋、皮蛋保存。

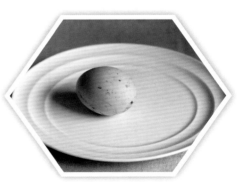

Ya Dan

Duck Egg

【Origin】
The egg of *Anas domstica* Linnaeus in the family of Anatidae.

【Collection / Processing】
Collect the duck eggs and use when they are fresh, or they can be processed into salty eggs or preserved eggs.

【Flavor / Properties】 Sweet in flavor and cold in nature.

【Meridian Tropism】 Lung and Large Intestine.

【Functions and Indications】
Nourish *yin*, clear the lung, and check diarrhea. Recommended for pyretic pulmonary patients with cough, or those with sore throat or pyretic diarrhea.

【Preparation / Consumption】
Boiled, braised, stir-fried, stewed, or fried. It can also be processed into salty eggs or preserved eggs.

【Cautions / Contraindications】
Large quantity of consumption is not recommended. Contraindicated for those with *yang* deficiency of the spleen, cold-damp diarrhea, or glomus and oppression due to *qi* stagnation after food.

【Storage】
Use fresh, or cold-stored in refrigerator, or preserved after being processed into salty egg or preserved egg.

鹌鹑蛋
An Chun Dan

【基原或来源】

　　为雉科动物鹌鹑 *Coturnix coturnix* Linnaeus 的卵。

【采收加工或制法】

　　取鹌鹑蛋鲜用。

【性味】味甘，性平。

【归经】入心、脾、胃经。

【功用】

　　补中益气、健脾益胃。适宜于体质虚弱，营养不良，气血不足，神经衰弱，心脏病者食用。

【服食方法】

　　可煮、炖、烧、炒等后食用。

【食宜食忌】

　　有痰饮、积滞及宿食内停者不宜多食。

【储藏】

　　鲜用，或宜冰箱中冷藏。

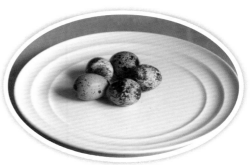

An Chun Dan

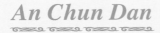

Common Quail Egg

【Origin】

The egg of *Coturnix coturnix* Linnaeus in the family of Phasianidae.

【Collection / Processing】

Collect the common quail eggs and use fresh.

【Flavor / Properties】 Sweet in flavor and neutral in nature.

【Meridian Tropism】 Heart, Spleen, and Stomach.

【Functions and Indications】

Strengthen the middle energizer and benefit *qi*, invigorate spleen and benefit stomach. Recommended for those with weakness, malnutrition, insufficiency of *qi* and blood, neurasthenia, or heart disease.

【Preparation / Consumption】

Boiled, braised, roasted, or stir-fried.

【Cautions / Contraindications】

Large quantity of consumption is not recommended for those with phlegm-rheum, dyspeptic disease and abiding food.

【Storage】

Use fresh, or kept in refrigerator.

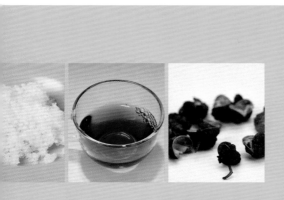

调味类
Seasonings

食 盐
Shi Yan

【基原或来源】

为海水或盐井、盐池、盐泉中盐水经煎炼或日晒而成的结晶体。

【采收加工或制法】

先经过晒或煮盐，待晶体析出，得到粗盐；再经溶解、沉淀、过滤、蒸发，制出精盐，加入碘者称为碘盐。一般超市均有袋装碘盐出售。

【性味】味咸、微辛，性寒。

【归经】入心、肺、肝、胃、肾、大肠经。

【功用】

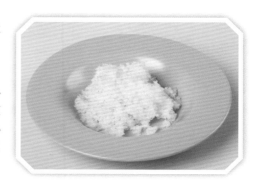

凉血解毒，涌吐壮骨。适宜于心腹痛，牙龈出血，宿食不化，胸中痰澼，皮炎，毒虫咬伤，疮疡肿痛，小便不通，便秘，视物不明，小儿疝气者使用。

【服食方法】

为凉菜、热菜、煲汤、做馅等的主要调味品，也是制作蔬菜或肉类腌制品的保鲜和调味辅料。

【食宜食忌】

高血压、肾病、咳嗽等患者慎食。

【储藏】

放入罐内或袋中密封，置于阴凉干燥处保存；防潮。

Shi Yan

Salt

【Origin】

Boil out of the sea water or saline water of salt well, pond or spring, or dry in the sun to form the crystals.

【Collection / Processing】

Dry the saline water in the sun or boil out the water to dissolve out the crystals thus get the crude salt. Then dissolve, deposit, filtrate, and evaporate the crude salt to get refined salt. If add iodine into the salt, it is known as the iodised salt, which can be bought in the supermarket.

【Flavor / Properties】 Salty and slightly pungent in flavor, cold in nature.

【Meridian Tropism】 Heart, Lung, Liver, Stomach, Kidney and Large Intestine.

【Functions and Indications】

Cool blood to detoxicate, promote emesis and strengthen bone. Used for chest and abdominal pain, gum bleeding, indigestion, turbid phlegm in chest, dermatitis, bites by noxious insects, ulcers, carbuncles and swellings, urinary obstruction, constipation, blurred vision, pediatric hernia, etc.

【Preparation / Consumption】

It is the main seasoning for cooking as well as for refreshing and processing vegetables and meats.

【Cautions / Contraindications】

The one who has hypertension, nephropathy and cough should take it with caution.

【Storage】

Preserved in a pot or bag air-tightly in cool and dry place and prevented from moisture.

酱
Jiang

【基原或来源】

为用大豆、麦子等做原料，经蒸罨发酵，并加入盐、水所制成的糊状食用物。

【采收加工或制法】

大豆酱制法：大豆7份、面粉3份、食盐1.7份、水10份。先拣除豆中杂质，洗净；再浸泡约10小时至大豆发胀；控除水后放入锅内煮2小时，再焖6～8小时，使豆呈黄褐色的糜糊状；将熟豆冷却至约37℃，与面粉拌匀，盖上净布密封，置于温度稍高处发酵；约7天后即可长出一层黄绿色毛，将其捣成小块，放于缸内，加入食盐与水，搅拌均匀，放于向阳处；约10天后，待酱呈红褐色，散发咸香之味时即可食用。

【性味】 味咸、甘，性冷。

【归经】 入肺、肾、大肠经。

【功用】

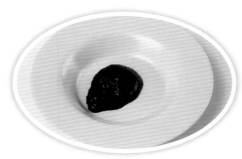

清热解毒，止血。适宜于燥热烦闷，中暑，瘟疫，烫伤，疥疮，鱼肉、蔬菜中毒，蛇、虫、犬咬伤毒，鸦片中毒，砒霜中毒，烟火毒，便秘，妊娠下血，尿血者使用。

【服食方法】

常作为凉拌菜、炒菜等的调味品食用；亦可用馒头、黄瓜、葱等蘸酱即食。

【食宜食忌】 小儿不宜多食；咳嗽、疖肿等患者慎食。

【储藏】

放瓶或罐内密封，置于阴凉处保存，防虫。

Jiang

Sauce

【Origin】

It is the edible paste which is evaporated and fermented with salt and water from soybean and wheat, etc.

【Collection / Processing】

It is made from soybean. It needs 7 shares of soya beans, 3 flour, 1.7 salts and 10 water.

【Flavor / Properties】 Salty and sweet in flavor, cold in nature.

【Meridian Tropism】 Lung, Kidney and Large Iintestine.

【Functions and Indications】

Clear heat and detoxicate, stop bleeding. Used for vexation due to dryness and heat, sun stroke, plague, scalding, scabies, food poisoning from flesh of fish or vegetables, bites by snakes, insects and dogs, opiumism, arsenic poisoning, fireworks poisoning, constipation, bleeding during pregnancy, hematuria, etc.

【Preparation / Consumption】

Usually used as cooking seasonings and it can be taken with steamed bread, cucumber and green onion.

【Cautions / Contraindications】

Children should not take it too much and the one who has cough, furuncles and swelling should take it with caution.

【Storage】

Preserved in a bottle or pot air-tightly in cool place and prevented from moth.

醋
Cu

【基原或来源】

为用米、高粱、玉米或酒、酒糟等为原料酿制而成的含有乙酸的液体；也有以食用冰醋酸加水、着色料配成的。现也有用各种水果或蔬菜酿醋。

【采收加工或制法】

选购时以颜色清凉，味酸而不涩、香而微甜，摇晃时有一层细小泡沫浮于上面，且持续较长时间者为佳。

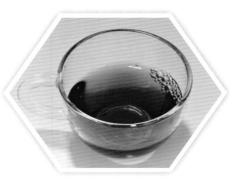

【性味】 味酸、甘、微苦涩，性温。

【归经】 入肝、胃经。

【功用】

消肿散瘀，益血开胃，解毒。适宜于癥瘕，食积，食欲不振，咽炎，黄疸，水肿，产后血晕，乳痈，血管硬化，高血压，疮痈肿毒，鱼肉菜毒者使用。

【服食方法】

常作为烹饪调味品，亦可兑热水饮用或制作饮料等。

【食宜食忌】

咳嗽、痢疾、牙齿不固的患者慎用。

【储藏】

放于瓶或罐内密封保存。

Cu

Vinegar

【Origin】

It is a kind of liquid containing acetic acid, which is made from rice, broomcorn, corn or brewed by the raw materials such as wine and distillers' solubles. It can also be made from edible glacial acetic acid with water and coloring materials. And there are various kinds of brewed vinegar made from fruits and vegetables.

【Collection / Processing】

The liquid with clear color, sour taste but not puckery, savoury and a little bit sweet, a layer of tiny bubbles when shaking the bottle and the bubbles can be lasted for a relativly long time is of good quality.

【Flavor / Properties】 Sour, sweet and slightly bitter in flavor, warm in nature.

【Meridian Tropism】 Liver and Stomach.

【Functions and Indications】

Relieve swelling and resolve stasis, benefit blood and improve appetite, detoxicate. Used for abdominal mass, indigestion and inappetence, pharyngitis, jaundice, edema, postpartum anemic fainting, acute mastitis, vascular sclerosis, hypertension, sores, carbuncles and pyogenic infections, food poisoning by fish, etc.

【Preparation / Consumption】

It is usually used as cooking seasonings or added in water for drinking. And it can be used to make drinks.

【Cautions / Contraindications】

The one who has cough, dysentery and unstable teeth should take it with caution.

【Storage】

Preserved in a bottle or pot air-tightly.

香 油
Xiang You

【基原或来源】

为胡麻科植物芝麻 *Sesamum indicum* DC. 的种子榨取的脂肪油。

【采收加工或制法】

秋季采收芝麻种子，晒干后选取质量上乘者炒熟后榨取油脂。炒时应掌握好火候和时间，避免炒熟过度影响榨出油的质和量。

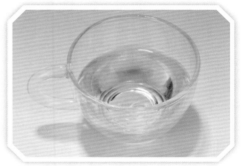

【性味】味甘，性凉。

【归经】入大肠经。

【功用】

解毒消肿，生肌止痛，润肠通便。适宜于肿毒初起，疮疡疼痛，疥癣，皮肤皲裂，蛔虫病，便秘，病后脱发，须发早白者使用。

【服食方法】

用于制作各种凉菜、菜馅、面食、糕点或炒菜时作调料食用。

【食宜食忌】

习惯性便秘者、老年人无脾胃虚弱者宜食。

【储藏】

置于阴凉处密封保存。

Xiang You

Sesame Oil

【Origin】

The fatty oil squeezed from the seeds of *Sesamum indicum* DC. in the family of Pedaliaceae.

【Collection / Processing】

Collect the sesame seeds in autumn, get them dried, and choose those with good quality to squeeze oil. When stir-frying, the flame and time need to be controlled to avoid influencing the quality and quantity of the oil because of excessive frying.

【Flavor / Properties】 Sweet in flavor and cool in nature.

【Meridian Tropism】 Large Intestine.

【Functions and Indications】

Subside swelling by resolving toxins, promote tissue regeneration and relieve pain, loosens bowel to relieve constipation. Recommended for those with initial swelling toxin, pain from sores ulceration, mange, skin chap, ascariasis, constipation, alopecia after disease, or premature graying.

【Preparation / Consumption】

It can be used to make various kinds of cold dishes, stuffing, cake, or as flavoring for cooking.

【Cautions / Contraindications】

Highly recommended for those with habitual constipation and the aged without weakness of the spleen and stomach.

【Storage】

Sealed up in shady area.

胡 椒
Hu Jiao

【基原或来源】

为胡椒科植物胡椒 *Piper nigrum* L. 干燥近成熟的果实（黑胡椒）或已除去外果皮的干燥成熟果实（白胡椒）。

【采收加工或制法】

每年的四、十月份，当果穗基部的果实开始变红时，剪下果穗，晒干或烘干后，即成黑褐色，取下果实，通称"黑胡椒"。如全部果实均已变红时采收，用水浸渍数天，擦去外果皮，晒干，则表面呈灰白色，通称"白胡椒"。除去杂质及灰屑，粉碎成细粉使用。

【性味】味辛，性热。

【功用】

温中止痛，散寒止泻，下气消积，祛痰解毒。用于风寒感冒，胃寒冷痛，反胃呕吐，泄泻冷痢，食欲不振，跌扑肿痛，药食阴毒。

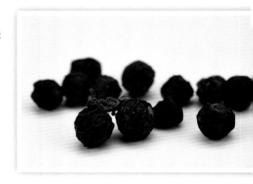

【服食方法】

作佐料，调味料食用。

【食宜食忌】

阴虚有火、内热素盛者忌食。

【储藏】

密闭，置阴凉干燥处保存。

Hu Jiao

Pepper

【Origin】

It is the dry and nearly mature fruit (black pepper) or the dry and nearly mature fruit without pericarp (white pepper) of *Piper nigrum* L. of the family Pipraceae.

【Collection / Processing】

In April and October each year, when the fruits begin to turn into red, cut the fruit cluster and have it dried. When it becomes black brown, collect the fruit and it is commonly called black pepper. If all the fruits have turned into red, soak them in water for some days and then remove the pericarp. The surface of the fruit without pericarp can become grey white after being dried, which is commonly called white pepper. Remove the impurities and grind them into powder.

【Flavor / Properties】 Pungent in flavor and hot in nature.

【Functions and Indications】

Warm the middle to arrest pain, disperse cold to stop diarrhea, drive *qi* downward to remove stagnation, and dispel phlegm to resolve toxins. It is used for treating common cold due to wind-cold, cold pain in the stomach, regurgitation, vomiting, diarrhea, cold dysentery, poor appetite, falls and knocks, swellings, and intake of *yin* toxins.

【Preparation / Consumption】

Can be served as seasoning.

【Contraindications / Cautions】

Not recommended for those with *yin* deficiency and excess internal heat.

【Storage】

Store in a sealed container and keep in a shady, cool and dry area.

花 椒
Hua Jiao

【基原或来源】

为芸香科植物花椒 *Zanthoxylum bungeanum* Maxim、青椒 *Zanthoxylum schinifolium* Sieb.et Zucc的成熟果皮。

【采收加工或制法】

8～10月果实成熟后，剪取果枝，摊开晾晒，待果实干裂，除净枝叶杂质，分出种子（椒目），取用果皮。

【性味】味辛，性温。有毒。

【归经】入脾、胃、肺、肾经。

【功用】

温中止呕，散寒止痛，降气止咳，除湿杀虫。用于脘腹冷痛，呕吐泄泻，咳嗽气逆，虫积腹痛，泄泻痢疾，阴痒疮疥。

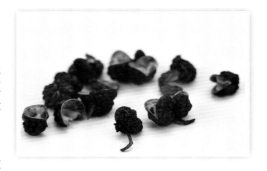

【服食方法】

可做调料或磨粉和盐拌匀为椒盐，供蘸食用。

【食宜食忌】

孕妇慎食；糖尿病等阴虚火旺者或肠热下血者忌食。

【储藏】

放置于密封干燥的容器中保存。

Hua Jiao

Pricklyash Peel

【Origin】

It is the mature pericarp of *Zanthoxylum bungeanum* Maxim or *Zanthoxylum schinifolium* Sieb.et Zucc of the family Rutaceae.

【Collection / Processing】

After the fruit is ripe from August to October, cut the fruit branch and dry it in the sun until the fruit cracks. Remove the impurities like branches, leaves and seeds and collect the pericarp.

【Flavor / Properties】 Pungent in flavor, warm in nature and toxic.

【Meridian Tropism】 Spleen, Stomach, Lung and Kidney.

【Functions and Indications】

Warm the middle to stop vomiting, disperse cold to stop pain, direct *qi* downward to treat cough, drains dampness and kills worms. It is used for treating cold pain in the abdomen, vomiting, diarrhea, cough, *qi* counterflow, abdominal pain due to intestinal worm accumulation, diarrhea, dysentery, vaginal itching and scabies.

【Preparation / Consumption】

Can be served as seasoning, or grinded into powder to mix with salt for dip.

【Contraindications / Cautions】

Use caution during pregnancy. Not recommended for those with *yin* deficiency resulting in vigorous fire like diabetes or bloody stool due to intestinal heat.

【Storage】

Store in a dry and sealed container.

红 糖
Hong Tang

【基原或来源】

为禾本科草本植物甘蔗 *Saccharum sinensis* Roxb. 的茎经压榨取汁炼制而成的赤色结晶体。

【采收加工或制法】

通俗方法常将甘蔗切碎碾压出汁液，先去除泥土、细菌、纤维等杂质，再以小火熬煮5~6小时，不断搅拌慢慢蒸发掉水分，使糖的浓度逐渐增高，待其冷却后凝固成为固体块状的红糖砖，再研磨成粉状即可。

【性味】 味甘，性温。

【归经】 入肝、脾、胃经。

【功用】

补脾和中，养血缓肝，活血祛瘀。适宜于瘀血内阻之产后恶露不尽，腹痛，月经不调，痛经，口干呕哕，年老体虚羸弱者使用。

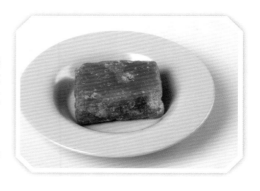

【服食方法】

入汤、作茶或溶化后服，亦可与黄酒、药汁同服。

【食宜食忌】

不宜多食、久食，不宜与鲫鱼、笋、葵等同食。体型偏胖、湿热内蕴、痰湿中阻者不宜食。糖尿病患者、高血脂患者等不宜食用。

【储藏】

置干燥容器内密封保存。

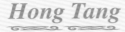

Hong Tang

Brown Sugar

【Origin】

It is the brown crystals which is processed from the squeezed juice of the stem of *Saccharum sinensis* Roxb. of family Gramineae.

【Collection / Processing】

Cut the sugarcane into pieces and squeeze juice. Remove the impurities such as soil, bacteria and fibers, stew the juice with soft fire for 5~6 hours and stir the liquid slowly to evaporate the moisture. Then the sugar concentration will gradually get high. At last, grind the congealed solid sugar brick into powder.

【Flavor / Properties】 Sweet in flavor and warm in nature.

【Meridian Tropism】 Liver, Spleen and Stomach.

【Functions and Indications】

Tonify spleen and harmonize the middle energizer, nourish blood and alleviate liver, activate blood to remove stasis. Used for endless postpartum lochia, abdominal pain, irregular menstruation, dysmenorrhea, dry mouth, vomiting, the sick and the old, etc.

【Preparation / Consumption】

Put into soup or tea to resolve the sugar, or take it with millet wine or decoction.

【Cautions / Contraindications】

It should not be taken too much or too long and it is unadvisable to take it with crucian, bamboo shoot or sunflower. Besides, the one who has a chubby body, internal dampness and heat, obstructed phlegm and dampness, diabetes, hyperlipidemia should not take it.

【Storage】

Preserved in a dry container air-tightly.

白砂糖
Bai Sha Tang

【基原或来源】

为禾本科植物甘蔗 *Saccharum sinensis* Roxb. 的茎汁，经精制而成的乳白色结晶体。

【采收加工或制法】

以甘蔗为原料，经提汁、清净、蒸发、结晶、分蜜和干燥等工序制作而成。

【性味】味甘，性平。无毒。

【归经】入脾、肺经。

【功用】

和中缓急，生津润燥。用于中虚腹痛，口干渴，燥咳。

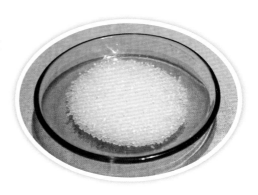

【服食方法】

入汤和化，做调味品。

【食宜食忌】

湿重中满者慎食，小儿忌多食。

【储藏】

放干燥、阴凉处保存。

Bai Sha Tang

White Granulated Sugar

【Origin】

It is the stem juice of *Saccharum sinensis* Roxb. of family Poaceae, which is refined as milky crystals.

【Collection / Processing】

Take the sugarcane as raw material, process it with juice extraction, lustration, evaporation, crystallization, honey separation and drying step by step.

【Flavor / Properties】 Sweet in flavor, moderate in nature and non-toxic.

【Meridian Tropism】 Spleen and Lung.

【Functions and Indications】

Harmonize the middle energizer to relieve spasm, generate fluid and moisten dryness. Used for abdominal pain due to deficiency of the middle energizer, dry mouth and thirst, dry cough.

【Preparation / Consumption】

Put it in the soup or make seasoning.

【Cautions / Contraindications】

The one who has abdominal distention due to over dampness should take it with caution and children should not take sugar too much.

【Storage】

Preserved in dry and cool place.

蜂 蜜
Feng Mi

【基原或来源】

为蜜蜂科蜜蜂属动物中华蜜蜂 *Apis carana* Fabr. 等所酿的蜜糖。

【采收加工或制法】

多在夏秋季采收，先将蜂巢割下，放于袋中再将蜜挤出即可。现超市皆有罐装品出售。

【性味】味甘，性平。

【归经】入肺、脾、胃、大肠经。

【功用】

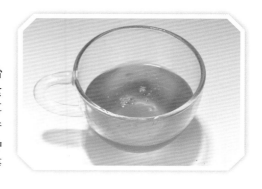

补脾润肺，止痛解毒。适宜于治脾虚无力，肺燥咳嗽，心烦意乱，食欲不振，阴虚内热，口渴，便秘，耳目失聪，惊悸失眠，肌肉疼痛，难产者使用。外用可治疗烫伤，疮疡肿毒，肌肤粗糙，口腔溃疡，牙龈炎等病症。

【服食方法】

可直接食用，或温开水冲服，煮粥，菜肴配料，制作蜜饯，酿酒，作为制作膏方的辅料，制作饮料等。

【食宜食忌】

素体痰湿者、呕吐者、饮酒过多者慎食。

【储藏】

放于罐内密封保存，防虫、防霉。

Feng Mi

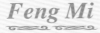

Honey

【Origin】

The honey brewed by *Apis carana* Fabr. of *Apis* genus in the family of Apidae.

【Collection / Processing】

Usually collected in summer or autumn. Cut the honey combs and put them into bags to extrude the honey. The canned honey can be easily found in common supermarkets.

【Flavor / Properties】 Sweet in flavor and neutral in nature.

【Meridian Tropism】 Lung, Spleen, Stomach and Large Intestine.

【Functions and Indications】

Invigorate the spleen and moisturize the lung, relieve pain and remove toxin. Used to resolve weakness due to spleen asthenia, cough due to lung dryness, distraction, poor appetite, intrinsic heat due to *yin* asthenia, thirsty, constipation, hearing and seeing loss, palpitation and insomnia, myalgia, and dystocia. For external use, it can be used to resolve scalding, swelling and toxin of sores, rough skin, mouth ulcer, and gingivitis.

【Preparation / Consumption】

It can be used directly, or mixed with warm water. It can also be made into porridge, used as cooking ingredients, made into preserved fruit, wine or beverages, and it can be used as adjuvant of Paste Formula.

【Cautions / Contraindications】

Use caution for those with phlegm-damp, vomiting, or excessive drinking.

【Storage】

Sealed air-tightly in vermins and mould proofing pots.

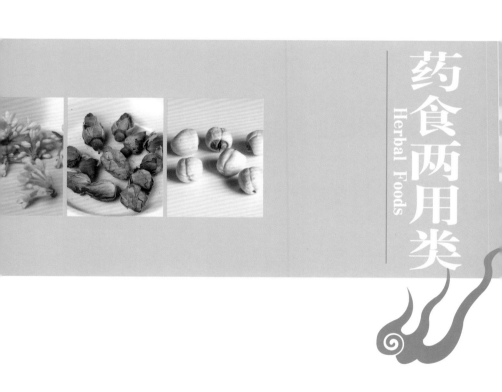

药食两用类
Herbal Foods

茶 叶
Cha Ye

【基原或来源】

　　为山茶科茶属植物茶 *Camellia sinensis*(L.) O. Ktze. 的嫩叶或芽。

【采收加工或制法】

　　春、夏季节采收初发的嫩叶或芽，尤以清明前后采收的嫩芽品最佳。少作鲜用，多干燥备用。

【性味】味苦、甘，性凉。

【归经】入心、肺、胃、肾经。

【功用】

　　清利头目，除烦止渴，消食化痰，利尿。适宜于热病心烦口渴，暑热，风热头痛，目赤昏花，消化不良，食积，口臭，小便不利、涩滞，多睡善寐者使用。

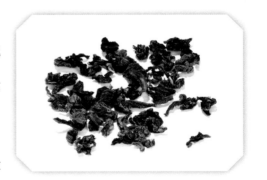

【服食方法】

　　泡饮，鲜嫩叶或嫩芽可烹饪时放入作调味用。

【食宜食忌】

　　失眠者不宜用；空腹、酒后、消化性溃疡者不宜多用、不宜浓茶、隔夜茶。不宜长期饮用浓茶。

【储藏】

　　干燥密封保存，防潮、防霉、防蛀。

Cha Ye

Tea Leaf

【Origin】
　　It is the tender leaves or buds of *Camellia sinensis*(L.) O. Ktze. of *Camellia* of family Theaceae.

【Collection / Processing】
　　Collect the incipient tender leaves and buds in spring and summer, especially the tender buds collected around Qingming are of good quality. Usually, the leaves are dried.

【Flavor / Properties】　Bitter and sweet in flavor, cool in nature.

【Meridian Tropism】　Heart, Lung, Stomach and Kidney.

【Functions and Indications】
　　Refresh head and eyes, relieve dysthesia and quench thirst, promote digestion and resolve phlegm, promote urination. Used for vexation and thirst due to febrile disease, summer heat, headache due to wind heat, hot eyes and blurred vision, poor appetite and indigestion, halitosis, difficult urination, drowsiness, etc.

【Preparation / Consumption】
　　Steep the dried leaves in boiling water or put the fresh tender leaves and buds in dishes when cooking as seasonings.

【Cautions / Contraindications】
　　It is not suitable for the insomniac. The one who has empty stomach and peptic ulcers or drinks should not take it too much or have strong tea and the tea of the previous night. It is unadvisable to have strong tea for long term.

【Storage】
　　Preserved air-tightly in dry container and prevented from moisture, mildew and moth.

茯苓
Fu Ling

【基原或来源】

为多孔菌科真菌茯苓 *Poria cocos* (Schw.) Wolf 的干燥菌核。

【采收加工或制法】

多于7~9月到马尾松林中采挖，堆置"发汗"后，摊开晾至表面干燥，再"发汗"，反复数次至现皱纹、内部水分大部散失后，阴干，称为"茯苓个"；或将鲜茯苓去皮后切制成块或片，阴干。

【性味】味甘、淡，性平，无毒。

【归经】入心、脾、肺、胃经。

【功用】

利水渗湿，健脾和胃，宁心安神。用于水肿胀满，小便不利，痰饮眩悸，脾虚泄泻，奔豚气逆，心神不安，惊悸失眠。

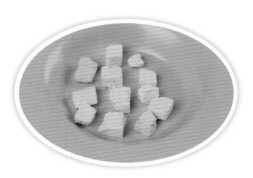

【服食方法】

煮粥或用于糕饼点心、饮料汤羹中。

【食宜食忌】

虚寒滑精或气虚下陷者慎用。

【储藏】

本品宜放置在阴凉干燥处，防潮、防冻、防热。

Fu Ling

Poria

【Origin】

It is the sclerotium of eumycete *Poria cocos* (Schw.) Wolf of the family Polyporaceae.

【Collection / Processing】

It is dug and collected in the masson pine forest in July to September each year. It is then packed together until fluid beads show on its surface. Spread them out until the surface is dried. Then pack them together again and repeat previous procedures for several times until it shows winkles and loses most of its internal moisture. Lastly, it is dried in shade. This is called 'individual poria'. Another processing is to cut fresh poria into slices or lumps and then dry them in the shade.

【Flavor / Properties】 Sweet, bland, neutral and non-toxic.

【Meridian Tropism】 Heart, Spleen, Lung and Stomach.

【Functions and Indications】

Induce diuresis and drain damp, invigorate spleen and harmonize stomach, calm the heart and mind. It is used for treating distention and fullness due to edema, difficult urination, vertigo due to phlegm rheum, diarrhea due to spleen deficiency, up-rushing of *qi*, mind restlessness, palpitations and insomnia.

【Preparation / Consumption】

Can be cooked into porridge or served as material in cakes, beverages and soups.

【Contraindications / Cautions】

Not recommended for those with seminal leakage due to cold deficiency or sinking of *qi* due to deficiency.

【Storage】

Stored in a shady, cool, and dry area. Contact with moist, frost and heat should be avoided.

桂 花
Gui Hua

【基原或来源】

为木犀科木犀属植物木犀 *Osmanthus fragrans* (Thunb.) Lour. 的花。

【采收加工或制法】

9~10月开花时采集，阴干备用。

【性味】味辛，性温。

【归经】入肺、肝、胃、大肠经。

【功用】

生津辟臭，散寒消瘀，化痰止咳。适宜于牙痛口臭，痰饮咳嗽，经闭腹痛，肠风血痢，疝疝奔豚等病症者使用。

【服食方法】

可泡茶，酿酒，制桂花露，盐渍，糖制，作糕点馅等。

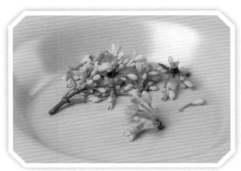

【食宜食忌】

阴虚火旺者慎食。

【储藏】

置于袋内密封保存。

Gui Hua

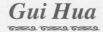

Osmanthus

【Origin】

It is the flower of *Osmanthus fragrans* (Thunb.) Lour. of *Osmanthus* of family Oleaceae.

【Collection / Processing】

Collect the flower in September and October, dry the flower in the shade for use.

【Flavor / Properties】 Pungent in flavor and warm in nature.

【Meridian Tropism】 Lung, Liver, Stomach and Large Intestine.

【Functions and Indications】

Generate fluid and avoid foul smell, disperse cold and resolve blood stasis, dispel sputum and relieve coughing. Used for toothache and halitosis, phlegm-fluid retention, coughing, abdominal pain due to amenorrhea, dysentery with blood due to intestine wind, abdominal lumps due to up-rushing *qi* etc.

【Preparation / Consumption】

Make tea, brew wine or osmanthus dew, processed with salt or sugar, make cakes, etc.

【Cautions / Contraindications】

The one who has *yin* deficiency and fire hyperactivity should take it with caution.

【Storage】

Preserved in a bag air-tightly.

金银花
Jin Yin Hua

【基原或来源】

为忍冬科植物忍冬 *Lonicera japonica* Thunb.、红腺忍冬 *Lonicera hypoglauca* Miq.、山银花 *Lonicera confusa* DC. 或黄褐毛忍冬 *Lonicera fulvotomentosa* Hsu et S.C.Cheng. 的花蕾或初开的花。

【采收加工或制法】

夏初当花含苞未放时采摘，晾晒或阴干。

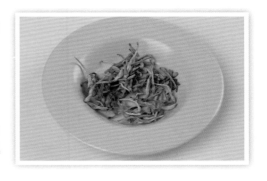

【性味】味甘、苦，性寒，无毒。

【归经】入肺、脾、胃经。

【功用】

清热解毒，疏散风热。用于疮疡肿毒，咽喉肿痛，热毒血痢，风热感冒，温病发热。

【服食方法】

鲜食干用均可，可调食，煮粥，泡茶，煎汤，捣汁，熬膏，制露等。

【食宜食忌】

脾胃虚寒者忌食。

【储藏】

干品置干燥容器内，防潮防蛀。

Jin Yin Hua

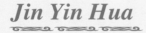

Honeysuckle

【Origin】

It is the Flower buds or the flower of initial blooming of *Lonicera japonica* Thunb., *Lonicera hypoglauca* Miq., *Lonicera confuse* DC., or *Lonicera fulvotomentosa* Hsu et S.C. cheng. of the family Caprifoliaceae.

【Collection / Processing】

It is collected before it blossoms in earlier summer. Dry it in the sun or in the shade.

【Flavor / Properties】 Sweet, bitter, cold and non-toxic.

【Meridian Tropism】 Lung, Spleen and Stomach.

【Functions and Indications】

Clear heat and resolve toxins, and disperse wind-heat. It is used for treating sores, swells, sore throat, bloody dysentery due to heat toxins, common cold due to wind-heat, fever due to warm disease.

【Preparation / Consumption】

It can be taken either fresh or dried. Can be mixed with other food, cooked into porridge, taken as tea, decocted with water, grinded for juice, made into paste or syrup, and so on.

【Contraindications / Cautions】

Not recommended for those with deficiency-cold of spleen and stomach.

【Storage】

The dry flowers should be stored in a dry container. Contact with moisture and insects should be avoided.

菊 花
Ju Hua

【基原或来源】

　　为菊科植物菊 *Chrysanthemum morifolium* Ramat. 的头状花序。

【采收加工或制法】

　　霜降前花正盛开时采收，晒干。

【性味】味甘、苦，性微寒，无毒。

【归经】入肺、肝经。

【功用】

　　散风清热，平肝明目，解毒消肿。平肝明目。适宜于风热感冒，头痛眩晕，目赤肿痛，眼目昏花，疗疮肿毒者食用。

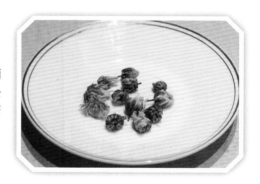

【服食方法】

　　泡茶，煮粥。

【食宜食忌】

　　脾胃虚寒者慎食。

【储藏】

　　可鲜用；阴干的菊花贮干燥容器内，置阴凉干燥处，防霉防蛀。

Ju Hua

Chrysanthemum

【Origin】

It is the capitulum of *Chrysanthemum morifolium* Ramat. of the Compositae family.

【Collection / Processing】

It is collected when flowers are in full blossoming before the Frost Descent (18th solar terms). The flowers are then dried in the shade.

【Flavor / Properties】 Sweet and bitter in flavor, slight cold in nature and non-toxic.

【Meridian Tropism】 Lung and Liver.

【Functions and Indications】

Disperse wind and clear heat, calm the liver and brighten the vision, remove toxin and subside swelling. It is used for treating common cold due to wind-heat, headache, dizziness, red, swell and painful eyes, blurred vision, boils and swells.

【Preparation / Consumption】

Can be taken as tea or cooked as a porridge.

【Contraindications / Cautions】

Not recommended for those with deficiency-cold of spleen and stomach.

【Storage】

It can be taken when it is fresh. The dried flowers should be stored in a dry container and in a shady, cool and dry area. Mould and contact with insects should be avoided.

玫瑰花
Mei Gui Hua

【基原或来源】

为蔷薇科植物玫瑰 *Rosa rugosa* Thunb. 和重瓣玫瑰 *Rosa rugosa* Thunb.f.plena (Regel)Byhouwer 的花蕾。

【采收加工或制法】

5、6月间采摘含苞未放的花朵，烘干或晒干。

【性味】味甘、微苦，性微温，无毒。

【归经】入肝、脾经。

【功用】

行气解郁，和血止痛。用于肝胃气痛，胃胀食少，月经不调，跌扑伤痛，新久风痹，消乳癖，痈肿，梅核气。

【服食方法】

煎汤、泡茶服、浸酒或熬膏用。

【食宜食忌】

阴血不足者慎用。

【储藏】

放密封器皿内，置阴凉干燥处保存。

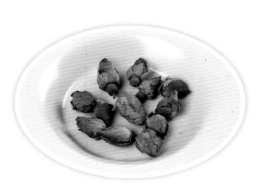

Mei Gui Hua

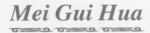

Rose

【Origin】

It is the flower bud of *Rosa rugosa* Thunb. and *Rosa rugosa* Thunb. f.plena(Regel)Byhouwer in the family of Rosaceae.

【Collection / Processing】

Pick the budding blossoms during May and June, dry the blossoms over a fire or in the sun.

【Flavor / Properties】 Sweet and slightly bitter in flavor, slightly warm in nature and non-toxic.

【Meridian Tropism】 Liver and Spleen.

【Functions and Indications】

Promote *qi* flow and resolve depression, harmonized blood and relieve pain. Commonly used for the one who has stomachache due to the attack of hyperactive liver-*qi*, bloated stomach and pool appetite, irregular menstruation, injuries from tumbles, new or old wandering arthritis, breast nodules, carbuncles and globus hystericus.

【Preparation / Consumption】

Cook soup, make tea, soak in wine or boil as paste.

【Contraindications / Cautions】

The one who is deficient in *yin* blood should take it with caution.

【Storage】

Preserved in the air-tight container and put it in the shady, cool and dry place.

茉莉花
Mo Li Hua

【基原或来源】

　　为木犀科植物茉莉 *Jasminum sambac* (L.) Ait. 的花。

【采收加工或制法】

　　7月前后花初开时，择晴天采收，晒干。

【性味】味辛、甘，性温。

【归经】入肝、脾、胃经。

【功用】

　　理气止痛，辟秽开郁，润燥香肌。适宜于湿浊中阻，胸膈不舒，泄泻痢疾，头晕目赤，皮肤干燥者使用。

【服食方法】

　　煮粥、代茶饮、制取花露等。

【食宜食忌】

　　火热内盛，燥结便秘者慎食。

【储藏】

　　贮存干燥处。

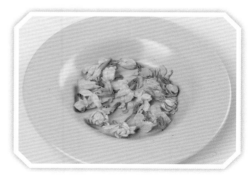

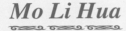
Mo Li Hua

Jasmine

【Origin】

It is the flower of *Jasminum sambac* (L.) Ait. of family Oleaceae.

【Collection / Processing】

Collect the flower in sunny days around July when it just blooms. Dry it in the sun.

【Flavor / Properties】 Pungent and sweet in flavor, warm in nature.

【Meridian Tropism】 Liver, Spleen and Stomach.

【Functions and Indications】

Regulate *qi* and relieve pain, prevent from the turbid and relieve depression, moisten dryness and perfume the skin. Used for turbid dampness obstructed in the middle energizer, discomfort of chest and diaphragm, diarrhea and dysentery, dizziness and pink eyes, dry skin.

【Preparation / Consumption】

Cook porridge, make tea or distill floral dew.

【Cautions / Contraindications】

The one who has excessive internal fire or constipation due internal dryness should take it with caution.

【Storage】

Preserved in dry place.

莲 子
Lian Zi

【基原或来源】

为睡莲科植物莲 *Nelumbo nucifera* Gaertn. 的成熟种子。

【采收加工或制法】

秋末、冬初割取莲房，取出果实，除去果皮，晒干，去心。

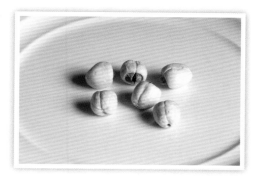

【性味】味甘、涩，性平，无毒。

【归经】入脾、肾、心经。

【功用】

健脾止泻，益肾涩精，养心安神。用于脾虚腹泻，下痢，梦遗滑精，虚烦失眠，崩漏带下，久痢下血，小便不禁。

【服食方法】

用来配菜、生食、蒸食、煮粥、做羹、炖汤、制饯、做糕点等。

【食宜食忌】

中满痞胀及大便燥结者忌食。

【储藏】

干品置干燥容器内，防霉，防蛀。

Lian Zi

Semen Nelumbinis

【Origin】

It is the ripe seed of *Nelumbo uncifera* Gaertn. of family Nymphaeaceae.

【Collection / Processing】

Cut the lotus seed pot during late autumn and early winter, take out the seed and peel off the seedcase, dry it in the sun and remove the plumule.

【Flavor / Properties】 Sweet and puckery in flavor, moderate in nature and non-toxic.

【Meridian Tropism】 Spleen, Kidney and Heart.

【Functions and Indications】

Invigorate spleen to check diarrhea, tonify kidney and secure essence, nourish heart and induce tranquilization. Commonly used for diarrhea due to spleen deficiency, nocturnal emission and spermatorrhea, dysphoria and insomnia, metrorrhagia and metrostaxis, morbid leucorrhea, long time diarrhea with blood and urinary incontinence.

【Preparation / Consumption】

Can be taken in the fresh form, or be used to make side dishes, steam, cook porridge, make thick soup, stew, make candy or desserts, etc.

【Contraindications / Cautions】

It is contraindicated for the one who has distention and fullness in the middle energizer and constipation.

【Storage】

The dried material should be preserved in dry container and prevented from the mildew and moth.